Psychology, Psychiatry and Chronic Pain

Psychology, Psychiatry and Chronic Pain

Edited by

Stephen P. Tyrer
Consultant Psychiatrist
Pain Relief Clinic
The Royal Victoria Infirmary
Newcastle upon Tyne, UK

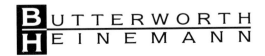

Butterworth-Heinemann Ltd
Linacre House, Jordan Hill, Oxford OX2 8DP

 PART OF REED INTERNATIONAL BOOKS

OXFORD   LONDON   BOSTON
MUNICH   NEW DELHI   SINGAPORE   SYDNEY
TOKYO   TORONTO   WELLINGTON

First published 1992

British Library Cataloguing in Publication Data
Psychology, Psychiatry and Chronic Pain
    I. Tyrer, Stephen P.
    616.89

ISBN 0 7506 0573 1

Typeset by Lasertext, Stretford, Manchester
Printed in Great Britain at the University Press, Cambridge

Contents

Contributors

P. Chandarana MB, ChB, ABPN, FRCP(C)
Associate Professor of Psychiatry, University of Western Ontario,
London, Ontario, Canada

J. E. Charlton MBBS, DObst, RCOG, FRCAnaes
Consultant Anaesthetist, Department of Anaesthesia, Pain Relief
Clinic, The Royal Victoria Infirmary, Newcastle upon Tyne, UK

P. T. James BSc, MPhil, CPsychol, AFBPsS
Department of Clinical Psychology, Pain Relief Clinic, The Royal
Victoria Infirmary, Newcastle upon Tyne, UK

G. Mendelson MBBS, MD, FRANZCP
Honorary Senior Lecturer, Monash University Department of
Psychological Medicine, Melbourne, Australia; and Consultant
Psychiatrist, Pain Management Centre, Caulfield General Medical
Centre, Caulfield, Victoria, Australia

H. Merskey DM, FRCP, FRCP(C), FRCPsych
Professor of Psychiatry, University of Western Ontario, London,
Ontario, Canada; and Director of Education and Research,
London Psychiatric Hospital, London, Ontario, Canada

L. M. Smith BSc (Hons), MCSP
Head of Therapy Services, West Dorset General Hospitals NHS
Trust

J. W. Thompson MBBS, PhD, FRCP
Director of Studies Honorary Physician, St. Oswald's Hospice,
Newcastle upon Tyne; Emeritus Consultant Clinical
Pharmacologist, Newcastle Health Authority; Emeritus Professor of
Pharmacology, University of Newcastle upon Tyne, UK

S. P. Tyrer MA, MB, BChir, LMCC, DPM, FRCPsych
Consultant Psychiatrist, Department of Psychiatry, Pain Relief
Clinic, The Royal Victoria Infirmary, Newcastle upon Tyne, UK

Foreword

This book is written in response to urgent needs at a time of growing crisis. The very phrase, chronic pain, merges in its meaning with intractable pain since neither condition would exist if safe powerful remedies were available. There are at least three reasons why the crisis grows. First, many of these pains occur in older people who make up a larger and larger fraction of our population, largely because of the success of the very same doctors who now fail to cure the pains of medically produced old age. Second, we have grown a community who no longer suffer in silence, and why should they be silent in a society which urges them to work, to be active and to participate. This means that private suffering is translated into public display which produces guilt and embarrassment in their friends and doctors who hide their impotence in a froth of frustration, anger and withdrawal. Third, and most peculiarly, the very real modern success in defeating certain types of pain emphasizes the pitiful failure of the cure of other types. We may tend to forget that there really have been huge successes for which those responsible should be very proud. Postoperative pain is an example of intelligent use of old recipes and of patient involvement and of new ideas which can transform a period of writhing discomfort into relative calm. The pains of terminal cancer have been abolished for the great majority of patients by the brilliant mobilization of humanity and thought over the past 50 years. Even as dramatic a condition as trigeminal neuralgia usually responds within a day to carbamazepine. One can therefore easily see the motivation of patients and professionals who now wish to advance from clear victories to conquer the remaining enemy.

First we must recognize how medicine has attacked a problem over the past 200 years. The first stage was to identify a causal pathology. Each disease was tracked down by the medicinal Sherlock Holmes to point a finger of accusation at the true criminal, be it bacterium, virus, cell, gene or molecule. In this Conan Doyle school of medicine, secondary characters were identified and placed on one side until the fundamental villain, the real Dr Moriarty, was nailed. In the eighteenth century, Heberden described a condition as precisely as any of us could do today but gave it the vague name of angina pectoris, pain in the chest. The reason for his vagueness was that he could not identify the causal local pathology. He examined the hearts of those who had died with extreme angina but he was not certain that he could detect a specific disorder of the heart to which he could ascribe the origin of the pain. We will return to Heberden's problems but, suffice it to say, over the next 200 years every structure in the chest; heart, lungs, blood vessels, nerves and joints, were labelled as the cause until, in the 1930s, P. D. White and Sir Thomas Lewis gave us the accepted explanation of today that ischaemic cardiac muscle causes angina pectoris. This set the scene for the doctors duty when faced with a patient in pain, which is to search for the pathology. They are very good at it. This patient has appendicitis. This patient has a broken leg. However there were serious problems which began to appear in this clearly successful process. Pain may not be associated with evident pathology. Certain types were so common that they could not be dismissed since even the doctors themselves suffered from them. The obvious example is the headache, subdivided into tension and migrainous types. Since they had to have a localized pathological cause the former was ascribed to muscle cramp and the latter to blood vessel dilatation or spasm. A hundred years on and it is now possible to measure with great precision the state of muscles and blood vessels and the fact that there is no correlation between these measurements and the headache has hardly dented the muscle tension and vascular origin dogma. Similarly, the ubiquitous back pain problems could be attributed to clear and classical spinal pathology; disc herniation, infection, tumour, stenosis, arthritis and arachnoiditis. In a larger and larger proportion of low back pain patients, none of these pathologies could be identified. Worse, a series of painful syndromes began to be identified for which the hard nosed could identify no pathology. These now include, temporomandibular joint syndrome, atypical facial neuralgia, whip lash syndrome, fibro-myalgia, repetitive strain syndrome, tenosynovitis, the majority of low back pain patients and post encephalitic myalgia.

Behind the honourable and successful search for localized pathological causes for abnormal symptoms, there was a more profound seventeenth century alternative. If someone reported a sensory experience which did not match the reality of the state of their body or the external world, they suffered a disorder of their mental world. This is Cartesian dualism in the raw. It is considered in every doctor's consultation room and in this book. Interestingly, Descartes himself was challenged by a Marquise with exactly this question when she asked him to explain a phantom limb. Descartes gave a much more subtle answer than many of those in this book who claim to be his loyal disciples. He explained that the mind was the slave of the body mechanisms and that the mind could not distinguish between a 'true' message and one delivered by a corrupted mechanism. This moves us 350 years on to understand a specific type of intractable pain where there has been obvious nerve damage in the periphery as in amputation, causalgia, Sudek atrophy, post herpetic neuralgia, arachnoiditis and spinal cord injury. If pain persists after all signs of the original peripheral damage has subsided, should we attribute the pain to a mental aberration as do some of the authors of this book or to the generation of 'false' signals as do others. The unravelling of this issue is exactly the crucial topic of this book. Of course the basic dualism of either body or mind may be incorrect since intermediate solutions to the question may be the most useful for those who suffer chronic pain.

Therefore let us leave the depths of these complex issues and return to the simple well known fact that abrupt cardiac ischaemia may produce a period of acute angina and death. There are also 'silent' fatal heart attacks where post mortem examination shows that a series of major unreported previous episodes of severe cardiac ischaemia had occurred. In patients with angina of effort, no clear correlation can be established between measured coronary circulation and angina. In the 1950s, 10 patients had sham operations and 10 had ligation of their internal mammary arteries for angina and both groups showed equal favourable pain responses over the next six months. Patients with osteoarthritis have clear precisely definable lesions of their joints and a limitation of movement and pain. The relation between these three is variable as is their response to joint replacement and to the many forms of drug treatment. These variations are the issues which make a book of this type so crucial for the future of our understanding of pain and, above all, for the well being of these patients.

We are hopefully beyond the crude dualism of the question 'Is it in the body or in the mind?' or in more fancy words, 'Is it sensory or affective?' or 'Is it real or cognitive-attentive-discriminative?' However, we may have to say to a patient 'I do not have the foggiest idea why you are in pain. You and I have to work on that question and in the meantime I have some useful things to tell you about how to live with this awful condition by teaching you methods of survival and coping and distraction and control.'

Patrick D. Wall FRS, DM, FRCP
Department of Anatomy and Developmental Biology
University College London, UK

Preface

Sufferers with chronic pain have a severe handicap to bear. Chronic pain is demoralizing and debilitating and it is not surprising that in this condition almost half of patients with chronic pain attending pain relief clinics have measurable psychiatric symptoms, mainly those of depression. Despite this, the majority of pain clinics do not have a regular service by psychologists or psychiatrists. There is more psychological input into pain clinics, but in the UK less than 5% of pain clinics have any dedicated sessions from psychiatrists.

This book is aimed at all those who work with individuals with chronic pain, so that they will be better able to assess and treat the psychological and psychiatric complications of this condition. It is not an academic textbook, rather it is intended to be a practical guide to help professionals not working in the mental health field about factors that affect the emotional state of chronic pain sufferers. It should therefore be of value to all doctors working with patients with chronic pain, to nurses, physiotherapists, occupational therapists, pharmacists, hypnotists and alternative therapists involved in this area. The psychologist or psychiatrist intending to work with patients with chronic pain and those who have some experience of the subject but wish more knowledge should also benefit from this volume. The intelligent pain sufferer should also find something of personal value from this work. The language used is intended to be free of jargon and should be understandable to the lay person.

The book is divided into two sections concerned with description of the issues involved in the psychological and psychiatric issues in chronic pain and in the second part, with assessment and intervention.

In addition to description of the main emotional factors involved in patients with chronic pain, there are chapters on particular psychiatric and psychological problems involved in specific illnesses and on compensation.

The second section on assessment and intervention describes what treatment methods are available to help those with emotional problems arising from chronic pain. There are chapters on psycho-tropic drugs, cognitive and behavioural therapy in chronic pain, and hypnosis. Chapters are also included on physiotherapy and the exhibition of transcutaneous electrical nerve stimulation (TENS) and acupuncture. A final chapter is concerned with how services can be organized within a chronic pain clinic.

A book with multiple authors from three different continents is difficult to organize in a comprehensive way. The fact that it has been achieved is in no small part due to the diligent attention of Vicky Woodruff, Gillian Simpson and Valerie Marsh who have together assembled the manuscript. Dr Trian Fundudis, Dr Marion Michie, Dr David Sanders and Dr Mark Tyrer have helped considerably in reading over selected passages in the book and offering valuable suggestions. Above all, I would like to thank my co-authors for their cooperation in assembling this volume. Finally, I am indebted to my wife who has put up nobly with my early morning risings and my evening irritability in order to get this work completed.

Stephen Tyrer
Newcastle upon Tyne

Part One

Descriptive Issues

1

Basic concepts of pain

S. P. Tyrer

The experience of pain is known to virtually all mankind. There are some people with certain neurological illnesses who are unable to feel pain but these are few and far between. So all of us, when describing and talking about 'pain', have a clear concept of what feeling is exhibited when we use the word. But do we? The experience of a sharp pain following a cut or burn is different in quality and description from the chronic, nagging pain of rheumatoid arthritis. The intermittent severe pain of gall-bladder colic, although incapacitating and intense when it occurs, does not have the long-term debilitating effects of the pain arising from chronic cancer or progressive arthritis. So each of us mean different things when we talk about pain and we cannot assume that others understand what we mean when we describe it.

The differences in the exhibition of pain described above are, to a large part, dependent upon the intensity and duration of the pain. In particular, chronic unremitting pain with little or no possibility of release must be one of the most distressing experiences known to man. The experience of pain dominates all waking life, it interferes with thinking and prevents all but the most simple of constructive activities. It disturbs sleep, impairs appetite, affects morale and may disorganize the functioning of every part of the body. It is largely with the problem of chronic pain that this book is concerned. Acute pain, although not free of psychological or psychiatric difficulties, is not usually associated with serious mental health effects.

Incidence

The incidence of chronic pain is enormous. In Britain about 2.2 million people a year see a doctor about a back problem. This is almost 5% of the adult population. However, the incidence of chronic backache at any one time is almost certainly higher than this. A survey population in Canada demonstrated a prevalence of 11% of the adult population with chronic pain and at any one time in the USA the percentage of adults with low back pain alone was found to be an extraordinarily high 17%.

In patients with psychological and psychiatric problems pain is frequently present and is also associated with psychological illness in patients seen in other medical disciplines. In general, over half of psychiatric outpatients spontaneously complain of pain during their illness. The incidence of pain in inpatients with psychiatric problems is somewhat less than this, at about 40%. A similar percentage of patients with pain arising from medical conditions have psychiatric problems. Pain and emotional illness are clearly closely related.

Definition of pain

With the increased realization that chronic pain has a different cause and course from acute conditions there have been changes in how pain has been defined. In prominent medical textbooks 20 years ago pain was defined simply as sensory experience caused by stimuli that injure. A large number of people with chronic pain show no objective evidence of present nerve or tissue damage and The International Association for the Study of Pain defined pain in 1979 as 'an unpleasant sensory and emotional experience associated with actual or potential tissue damage, or described in terms of such damage'. The group that made this definition emphasized that pain is always something that is individual to the sufferer. It is nearly always unpleasant and, like all unpleasant experiences, it has emotional consequences.

Many people with chronic pain are reluctant to see psychiatrists and psychologists in connection with their pain. They assume that if someone has referred them to somebody normally involved in the treatment of mental health problems that the belief is that they are imagining their pain and it must be in the mind. In fact, pain is always perceived at a conscious level and so must be 'in the mind'. The sufferer believes that if no evidence of damage to the body is found then the apparent sensation of pain must be imaginary. The succeeding chapters in this book will illustrate that this is not the case. A large number of experiences, stimuli and attitudes affect our perception of pain but it is never imaginary. Of more importance, psychological and psychiatric management techniques can help the sufferer to cope with pain whatever its origin.

For the purpose of this book, pain is considered to be an unpleasant experience. It is possible to weakly stimulate the nerves that carry pain messages and produce tingling or non-painful pain sensations. These experiences do not have unpleasant emotional consequences and so are not relevant to this text.

In another context, there are certain individuals who seem to get enjoyment from pain. These are described as masochistic people. Perhaps pain is pleasurable for these individuals? Masochistic behaviour is much rarer than one would imagine from reading novels and magazines and essentially involves the individual wishing to be humiliated. The infliction of pain is one way of doing this but is by no means the only method. Promoting *chronic* pain in this context is unusual and is more likely to be due to faulty technique than deliberate policy.

Anatomy of pain

Pain is usually caused by injury or inflammation and it is important for sense organs in the body that are affected by these changes to inform the brain as rapidly as possible what is occurring. The sensory units in the body that are able to detect injury should respond as quickly as possible to meet the danger of the noxious stimulus. On touching a red-hot poker there is reflex withdrawal of the hand away from the place of injury that occurs before the brain is aware of a problem. This withdrawal can occur without pain being felt. It is for this reason that the sensory units involved in detecting such stimuli are called nociceptors (i.e. noxious sensation receptors) rather than pain receptors.

All nerves consist of neurones or nerve cells that have long filaments called axons. Nociceptors are a specialized form of nerve cell that are found in all parts of the body but which are particularly concentrated in the skin and areas of the body that are exposed to possible injury. The classification of neurones is made entirely on the speed of conduction of nervous impulses. This depends on two factors: the diameter of the axon and myelination. Myelin consists of fatty material which ensheaths the nerve and acts as an electrical insulator enabling transmission of nervous impulses to take place more rapidly. The greater the degree of myelination the faster the speed of conduction. In addition, axons of larger diameter conduct faster than axons that are smaller, independent of the degree of myelination.

Types of nerves

Nerve fibres are designated from A to D according to their speed of conduction. The A fibres are the most rapidly conducting fibres and are further subdivided into alpha, beta, gamma and delta. A delta (A_δ) neurones are largely responsible for the rapid transmission of impulses to the brain that give rise to the sharp element of acute pain. A beta (A_β) neurones largely inhibit painful sensations. These fibres also respond to strong pressure but do not respond to heat or irritant chemicals unless damage is very severe. Injury from these sources is detected by smaller, unmyelinated C fibres. Transmission of information by these fibres is much slower than along the A_δ axons, about one metre per second as opposed to 10–25 metres per second for A_δ fibres.

This information helps to explain the sequence of events that occurs when touching a red-hot object. After withdrawal of the hand from the painful object there is a sharp pain followed by a persistent dull burning pain. The former pain arises from A_δ neurones, the second, longer-lasting pain is transmitted by C neurones. The nociceptors of the C group of neurones also become more sensitive to further stimulation after damage and this contributes to the tenderness and prolonged pain for a short period after even mild injuries.

Both the A_δ and C fibres terminate in the dorsal horn of the spinal cord. Their paths then diverge. Electrical activity cannot be transferred directly from one nerve to another. Instead a chemical substance, a neurotransmitter, is released from the nerve terminal in the immediate vicinity of the target neurone. This binds to receptors on the nerve membrane and so excites or inhibits the target neurone. Many transmitters also facilitate or modulate the effects of other neurotransmitters. The structural specializations associated with this process are called synapses and it is usual to distinguish neurones in a circuit relative to particular synapses. Thus a neurone may be termed a presynaptic or postsynaptic neurone.

The postsynaptic neurone involved in the transmission of fast nerve transmission (A_δ fibres) has an axon which crosses from the dorsal horn over the spinal cord in front of the central canal and runs in a collection of similar fibres (axons) or tract, to the thalamus, the first structure in the brain to process nociceptive information. The tract is called the lateral spinothalamic tract (Figure 1.1). Other A_δ fibres ascend to the reticula formation in the brain stem via the spinoreticular tract.

The more numerous C fibres also reach the brain but in a less direct way. They ascend as a series of short connecting neurones, with repeated synapses, before eventually reaching the thalamus or reticular formation in the brainstem. From here there is transmission to all parts of the cerebral cortex including the limbic system, the part of the brain that is concerned with emotion. When the nerve pathways between the thalamus and the limbic system are cut, pain is still appreciated but the associated emotions are diminished or lost. Finally, many of the fibres concerned with carrying pain information terminate in the cerebral cortex. The cortex enables the actual site of pain to be located with precision.

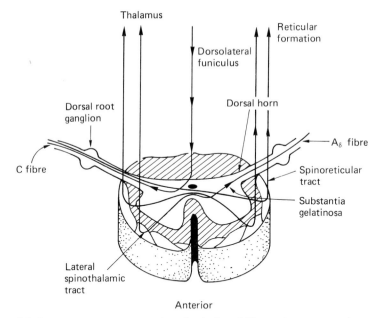

Figure 1.1 *Diagrammatic representation of spinal cord illustrating nerve tracks carrying pain fibres and their connections.*

The gate theory

For years there has been debate whether pain is a specific sensory phenomenon with its own particular receptors or whether it results when any stimulus is sufficiently intense to activate the receptors in the area affected. It is now felt that there is some truth in both these theories. It is known that emotion affects considerably the experience of pain. In 1965 Professor Melzack of Montreal and Professor Wall of London together proposed the Gate Theory to explain on physiological grounds how these factors could both affect the experience of pain. In principle, Melzack and Wall said that the information resulting from painful stimuli is altered in its passage from peripheral nerves to the spinal cord. This is achieved by the mechanism of a 'gate' situated in the dorsal horn of the spinal cord. The degree of pain perceived by the brain depends on how far the gate is open. There is now evidence for the neural basis of such a gate.

Transmission of information about pain to the brain depends upon activation of cells in the dorsal horn of the spinal cord called transmission (T) cells. These cells are influenced by both myelinated and unmyelinated fibres; the larger, myelinated fibres inhibit T cell transmission whilst the smaller, unmyelinated C fibres facilitate it. Activity in these nerve fibres depends in turn on the action of a further cell close by the spinal cord. This cell, called the substantia gelatinosa

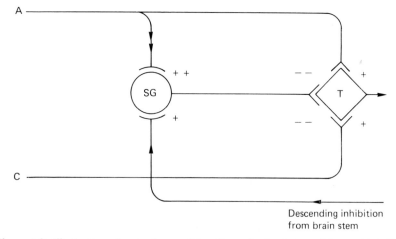

Figure 1.2 *Illustration of gate theory. The effect of stimulation of large (A$_\beta$) fibres and that of descending cortical influences is shown.*

cell (SG cell), because it is situated in part of the spinal cord called the substantia gelatinosa, is itself activated by branches from large myelinated fibres concerned with touch and proprioception and is inhibited by activity of the C fibres (Figure 1.2). The greater the activity of the SG cell the more T cell transmission is inhibited. There is normally activity in the C fibres but this is not sufficient to overcome the inhibition of the larger fibres.

When injury or inflammation results there is stimulation of receptors concerned with both touch and pain. The stimulation of the large fibres at first inhibits discharge of the T cell by activating the SG cell but eventually the T cell is activated by A$_\delta$ and C fibre transmission and the gate is opened allowing pain impulses to reach the brain. It can be seen that anything which stimulates the large fibres concerned with touch, pressure or temperature can inhibit T cell transmission and reduce the amount of pain perceived by the brain. This is the basis of the time-honoured remedy of rubbing the adjacent skin following an injury in order to reduce pain. Similarly, applying a cool dock leaf reduces the pain that results from being stung by nettles; although there is also a neurochemical mechanism involved here.

The T cell is also influenced by the state of mind of the individual. If the subject is relaxed and unworried, descending impulses from the dorsolateral funiculus activate the SG cell and inhibit T cell transmission. Conversely, when anxiety is high impulses pass down the spinal cord from the limbic system and activate the T cell, allowing increased perception of pain. However, some arousal states can be associated with decreased perception of pain suggesting that other factors close the gate in these instances.

Physiology of pain

To understand further the mechanisms involved in pain in these circumstances we need to know more about the identity of the neurotransmitters involved in pain and how these are related to pain perception.

Neurotransmitters involved in pain

The main neurotransmitters involved in those nerves concerned with the transmission of pain sensations are substance P, enkephalins, endorphins and serotonin. Other chains of amino acids called polypeptides similar to substance P, e.g. calcitonin-gene-related peptide, are also found in tissues in which sensory stimulation is usually painful, suggesting that these peptides are involved in the neurotransmission of painful impulses.

Substance P is a peptide that is found in the dorsal horn of the spinal cord in regions where many C fibres terminate. Since these fibres are implicated in the transmission of pain it seems probable that substance P is one of the main transmitters concerned in relaying pain messages. To understand how substance P is concerned in pain we need to know more about how neurotransmitters are involved in the transmission of pain messages. Although, in general, neurotransmitters are excitatory or inhibitory a large part of their actions are concerned with the modulation of the effects of other neurotransmitters at synapses. Thus, in the dorsal horn of the spinal cord we find substance P, which facilitates T cell transmission, opens the gate and increases pain. In the same area other neurotransmitters called enkephalins are found that modulate the effects of substance P and consequently tend to close the gate and reduce pain. Enkephalins are also found in other parts of the brain where substance P is present, particularly in the lower brainstem.

The enkephalins have similar properties to those of morphine, an opioid peptide. They produce analgesia, and a mild degree of euphoria as well as causing nausea, reducing activity of the gastrointestinal tract and depressing respiration. A similar substance produced by the pituitary gland called β-endorphin has also been found to reduce pain and antagonize the action of substance P. β-endorphin is much longer acting than the enkephalins and is probably released during high arousal and may account for the absence of pain in people who sustain injuries during intense physical activity. We also know that in certain pain-relieving procedures such as acupuncture, β-endorphin activity is increased.

Serotonin (or 5-hydroxytryptamine) is one of the monoamine group of neurotransmitters. The chief monoamines involved in neurotransmission are serotonin, dopamine and noradrenaline. Enkephalins activate neurones concerned with transmission of serotonin and when the levels of serotonin are increased, e.g. by giving an amino acid called L-tryptophan, analgesia occurs. Substances which increase dopamine also increase analgesia whereas depletion or blocking of amine receptor sites reverses this process.

Chemicals released by injury

Injury releases a number of chemicals which are involved in the production of pain. These substances are produced by damaged cells and stimulate the neurones. We know that long-chain fatty acids called prostaglandins are produced when tissue is damaged but other substances like histamine and potassium are probably also involved. In addition, injury causes peptides known as kinins to be formed in the blood and these can both produce pain directly and increase sensitivity to harmful stimuli. With increased knowledge about these factors it is possible to interrupt and antagonize the effects of pain. For instance, aspirin is a prostaglandin inhibitor and is probably effective in pain relief because of this mechanism.

Relevance of these mechanisms in chronic pain

The description of the anatomy and physiology of pain given above is largely applicable to pain arising from acute tissue damage. This type of pain is much easier to examine experimentally than chronic, persistent pain. Patients with chronic pain have a low tolerance to pain and also complain of poor sleep and appetite, irritability, constipation, fatigue and they are inclined to withdraw from others. We know the physiological basis of some of these symptoms but others are not clearly established and are generally labelled as having a psychological cause. However, all psychological events must ultimately have a physiological basis. In any case if no physical cause can be detected for the complaint of pain this does not automatically mean that it is psychological. Most patients have evidence of both physical and psychological contributions to their pain complaint.

It cannot be emphasized too highly that the relationship between the complaint of pain in patients with chronic pain is quite unrelated to tissue injury. Most studies actually show that patients with little to no evidence of pathological (organic) damage complain of higher degrees of pain that those with clear signs of injury.

In the vast majority of these cases the patients are suffering as much or even more than patients with a definite physical aetiology for their symptoms. In many of these cases, the original physical cause of their pain has disappeared but there are secondary pains arising because of lack of use of the affected part. If any part of the body is not utilized, particularly muscles and joints, there is shortening of muscle fibres and supporting structures and movement of the affected part causes pain. This pain is often perceived erroneously by the patient as due to the original damage which caused pain in the first place and further activity is avoided.

There is another reason why patients who have persistent pain complain of more severe symptoms. In experimental animals, a few days after sensory nerve damage, cells that previously responded to stimuli within their appropriate anatomical segment begin to respond to stimuli from other areas. Persistent electrical stimulation of C fibres in the rat lowers the threshold of the associated neurones and those that originally only responded to pinch start to respond to touch. The result of persistent nociceptive stimulation is both an increase in sensitivity of the receptors and an expansion of their receptive fields so that distant nociceptors are more likely to be excited.

Patients with chronic pain often have associated disabilities because of these factors which prevent them from taking part in activities in which they formerly used to take pleasure. There is increasing evidence that participation in pleasurable activities reduces pain by stimulating the production of endorphines and possibly enkephalins. Other factors, including past memory of painful events and response to painful experiences in the past will also influence the exhibition of and maintenance of behaviour associated with chronic pain. These issues are discussed in more detail in Chapters 10 and 11.

Measurement of pain

It should be clear by now that the relationship between painful stimulation and pain experience is not close, especially in patients with chronic pain. It is therefore not valuable to measure the degree of pain by recording the rate of transmission along the axons of C and A_δ neurons. Pain cannot be perceived until these impulses reach the brain and as the gate theory postulates it is the activation of the T cell which determines whether or not peripheral painful impulses reach consciousness. Theoretically, it should be possible to detect nervous impulses in the ascending nerves from the dorsal horn of the spinal cord to the brainstem, but even if this was practical, which it is not at present, there would almost certainly be a poor correspondence between the measurements obtained and the subject's description of the intensity and quality of his pain. The measurement of pain must therefore depend upon accurate descriptions by the subject of either existing pain, or of experimentally-produced pain. Even then, we are dependent upon the informant's ability to communicate and desire to do so. If a subject wishes to exaggerate or diminish the intensity of painful stimulation he or she will be able to do this successfully to a very large extent.

It is also essential to describe exactly what is meant when one is measuring pain. There are four levels at which pain can be assessed: the neurophysiological, perceptual, evaluative and behavioural. Most attention has been focused on the measurement of specific painful events.

When an unpleasant stimulus is applied there is a level at which the perception of this stimulus is evaluated as pain. This is the pain perception threshold and is normally constant in the same individual from one moment to the next. If an experimental painful stimulus is applied with increasing severity there comes a point when the subject perceives the pain as unbearable. The interval between the threshold for pain perception and that of severe pain is a measure of the subject's pain tolerance. The degree of pain tolerance varies widely between one individual and the next according to personality, cultural differences and mental state. People who are extrovert and outgoing have higher pain thresholds than introspective, introverted individuals. Those who are preoccupied with their health and, in particular, are concerned that they might have some serious physical disease, have a lower degree of pain tolerance than average. The culture from where the subject comes also has a bearing upon pain expression. The British psychologist, McDougall, showed as long ago as 1901 that islanders from New Guinea had higher thresholds for severe pain than British men. People from eastern cultures have higher tolerances for pain than those from the west. Anxiety and stress lower thresholds to pain, although certain forms of severe stress can actually relieve pain, possibly because β-endorphins are released.

Measurement of pain tolerance

The original experiments by McDougall involved the use of a weighted pointed object and the threshold of pain was reported in terms of kilograms of pressure on the thumb-nail, forefinger and forehand. This test is difficult to standardize and in 1965, Richard Sternbach, an American psychologist, devised a method for measuring pain tolerance by cutting off the blood supply to the arm. When muscles are deprived of their blood supply they become painful.

In Sternbach's tourniquet test the subject first raises his arm above his head, a blood pressure cuff is then applied around the upper arm and maintained at a pressure above that of the systolic blood pressure of the patient. This means that blood is unable to enter the arm through the arteries and pain will eventually result from the ischaemic muscles. After applying the tourniquet the patient squeezes a hand exerciser 20 times and the time recorded from cessation of this activity to the perception of unbearable pain is recorded. In a subject with chronic pain the extent of this can be experimentally determined by asking the subject to indicate at what time after the application of the tourniquet is the degree of pain equivalent to his present pain. The Tourniquet-pain ratio (TPR) can then be calculated according to the following formula:

$$TPR = \frac{\text{time to reach maximum pain tolerated}}{\text{time to reach intensity of present pain}} \times 100.$$

Another test that has been used for the same purpose involves immersing the forearm in ice-cold water. The time taken for pain sensations to be felt and ultimately very severe pain to occur can be recorded in the same way as for the Tourniquet test.

Self-assessment of pain

The above tests require an experimenter to apply a stimulus in order to measure the degree of pain. It is helpful to record the level of pain at other times without the intervention of another. One of the simplest ways of doing this, which is also one of the most accurate, is by means of what was originally described as the Pain Line. A diagrammatic representation of a Pain Line in use at the Newcastle Pain Relief Clinic is indicated in Figure 1.3.

The subject is asked to record the extent of their present pain by drawing a vertical line to intersect the Pain Line above. If, for example, the subject believes that their pain at present is 70% as bad as it could be they will apply their vertical mark 7 cm along the line from the left-hand point. This score is recorded and can be compared with the scores in the same patient at other times in the past. This can be very useful in evaluating the effect of different treatments and factors affecting pain.

Despite its simplicity, this scale is more accurate than verbal scales that use adjectives like mild, moderate and severe to describe pain. It is essential that the subject understands the principle of the test before being asked to carry out the instructions. In properly informed intelligent patients this test is highly accurate at determining *present* pain. More errors result when estimates of past pain are made. It is known that pre-existing pain affects judgement about past pain. When subjects are in severe pain they evaluate past pains as more severe than when their present pain is only mild. The converse also holds— patients with little or no known pain tend to underestimate the degree of previous pain experiences.

An estimate of the degree of pain experienced by different subjects

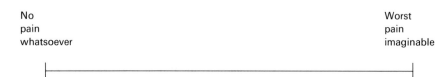

No   Worst
pain   pain
whatsoever   imaginable

Please indicate your present
degree of pain by making
a vertical mark on the
above line

Figure 1.3 *Visual analogue scale of pain measurement.*

can also be made by asking them to compare their present or past
pains with known painful conditions such as toothache, gall-bladder,
colic or a fractured limb. Even if subjects have not experienced these
conditions it has been found that they can estimate surprisingly
accurately the degree of pain that they cause, and this can be used to
determine the extent of present and past pain.

All these tests measure the intensity of pain. However, pain is not
just experienced as a sensation, but also in terms of its emotional
impact and what it means to the person concerned. In order to
measure these other aspects of pain, Professor Melzack and his
colleagues from Montreal designed a questionnaire called the McGill
Pain Questionnaire to examine the words that people use when
describing their painful experiences. Words like stinging and squeezing
describe sensory aspects of pain whereas adjectives like frightful and
wretched are more concerned with the emotional impact of the pain
on the sufferer. Words like troublesome indicate the intensity of pain
experienced. Subjects with anxiety and depression are more likely to
use words describing emotional aspects of pain than those describing
its sensory qualities. In addition, the questionnaire can be used to
measure the degree of pain and the changes in this over time, with
particular regard to whether changes have occurred in the sensory or
affective (mood) components of pain. Despite appearing cumbersome,
the McGill Pain Questionnaire is widely used and no alternative
questionnaire or schedule has been found to take its place.

The measurement of pain is an imprecise science and both self-evaluative and objective assessments are affected considerably by the patient's emotional state, past experience and duration of pain. However, as pain is an entirely subjective phenomenon this is to be expected. The interpretation of the measurements obtained with these methods is coloured by psychological and psychiatric factors. Assessment of these contributions to chronic pain is considered in Chapter 7.

Bibliography

Basbaum, A. T. and Fields, H. L. (1984) Endogenous pain control mechanisms: Review and hypothesis. *Annals of Neurology*, **4**, 451–462

Kerr, F. W. L. (1976) The ventral spinothalamic tract and other ascending systems of the ventral funiculus of the spinal cord. *Journal of Comparative Neurology*, **159**, 335–356

Wall, T. D. (1989) The dorsal horn. In *Textbook of Pain* (eds P. D. Wall, R. Melzack and J. J. Bonica), Edinburgh, Churchill Livingstone

2

Classification of pain

S. P. Tyrer

The classification of painful states is still in its infancy. The first attempt to classify all conditions with chronic pain was made in 1986 (IASP Sub-committee on Taxonomy) but as with all new systems a number of radical changes have since been proposed. The separation of emotional factors that contribute to chronic pain has been attempted as a separate exercise and this chapter will be concerned with the different systems that are at present in operation. All the systems described below are concerned with chronic pain, defined as pain that persists after the normal time for healing and which is present for at least six months.

There are three main classification systems that are used for categorizing psychological and psychiatric problems in chronic pain. These are:

1 The International Association for the Study of Pain (IASP) Taxonomy

2 *The Diagnostic and Statistical Manual,* 3rd edition, revised (DSM-III (R))

3 *The International Classification of Diseases,* 9th edition (ICD-9).

The ICD classification is being revised and a tenth edition is due shortly.

The main features of these three systems are indicated in Tables 2.1, 2.2 and 2.3. No one of these three systems is satisfactory on its own for the accurate classification of emotional factors in chronic pain although there are some advantages in all three systems. The problem with all of them is that they are too restrictive. A meaningful classification of psychological and psychiatric problems in chronic pain should include details about the cause of the condition, its ultimate outcome and the effects of specific treatment. Although in many cases these details are not known for chronic pain conditions the existing schemas are not sensitive enough to distinguish between patients with different causes for their pain and with varying emotional reactions. However, the existing classifications are better than none and are accepted by other workers in the field.

Table 2.1 International Association for the Study of Pain Sub-committee on Taxonomy Classification of Chronic Pain

Muscle tension pain

Delusional or hallucinatory pain

Hysterical or hypochondriacal pain

    Monosymptomatic, associated with emotional conflict
    Multiple complaints in addition to those of pain
    Hypochondriacal with preoccupation with somatic health

Table 2.2 DSM-III-R Classification of Chronic Pain

Somatoform Pain Disorder 307.80

A. Preoccupation with pain for at least six months.

B. Either (1) or (2):

    (1) appropriate evaluation uncovers no organic pathology or pathophysiologic mechanism (e.g. a physical disorder or the effects of injury) to account for the pain

    (2) when there is related organic pathology, the complaint of pain or resulting social or occupational impairment is grossly in excess of what would be expected from the physical findings.

Hypochondriasis (or Hypochondriacal Neurosis) 300.70

A. Preoccupation with the fear of having, or the belief that one has, a serious disease, based on the person's interpretation of physical signs or sensations as evidence of physical illness.

B. Appropriate physical evaluation does not support the diagnosis of any physical disorder that can account for the physical signs or sensations or the person's unwarranted interpretation of them *and* the symptoms in A are not just symptoms of panic attacks.

C. The fear of having, or belief that one has, a disease persists despite medical reassurance.

D. Duration of the disturbance is at least six months.

E. The belief in A is not of delusional intensity, as in Delusional Disorder, Somatic Type (i.e. the person can acknowledge the possibility that his or her fear of having, or belief that he or she has, a serious disease is unfounded).

Somatization Disorder 300.81

A. A history of many physical complaints or a belief that one is sickly, beginning before the age of 30 and persisting for several years.

(*continued*)

Table 2.2 *continued*

B. At least 13 symptoms from the list below. To count a symptom as significant, the following criteria must be met:

(1) no organic pathology or pathophysiologic mechanism (e.g. a physical disorder or the effects of injury, medication, drugs, or alcohol) to account for the symptom or, when there is related organic pathology, the complaint or resulting social or occupational impairment is grossly in excess of what would be expected from the physical findings.

(2) has not occurred only during a panic attack

(3) has caused the person to take medicine (other than over-the-counter pain medication), see a doctor, or alter life-style

Symptom list:

Gastrointestinal symptoms:

(1) **vomiting (other than during pregnancy)**
(2) abdominal pain (other than when menstruating)
(3) nausea (other than motion sickness)
(4) bloating (gassy)
(5) diarrhea
(6) intolerance of (gets sick from) several different foods

Pain symptoms:

(7) **pain in extremities**
(8) back pain
(9) joint pain
(10) pain during urination
(11) other pain (excluding headaches)

Cardiopulmonary symptoms:

(12) **shortness of breath when not exerting oneself**
(13) palpitations
(14) chest pain
(15) dizziness

Conversion or pseudoneurologic symptoms:

(16) **amnesia**
(17) **difficulty in swallowing**
(18) loss of voice
(19) deafness
(20) double vision
(21) blurred vision
(22) blindness
(23) fainting or loss of consciousness
(24) seizure or convulsion
(25) trouble walking
(26) paralysis or muscle weakness
(27) urinary retention or difficulty urinating

(continued)

Table 2.2 *continued*

Sexual symptoms for the major part of the person's life after opportunities for sexual activity:

(28) **burning sensation in sexual organs or rectum (other than during intercourse)**
(29) sexual indifference
(30) pain during intercourse
(31) impotence

Female reproductive symptoms judged by the person to occur more frequently or severely than in most women:

(32) **painful menstruation**
(33) irregular menstrual periods
(34) excessive menstrual bleeding
(35) vomiting throughout pregnancy

Note: The seven items in bold may be used to screen for the disorder. The presence of two or more of these items suggests a high likelihood of the disorder.

Undifferentiated Somatoform Disorder 300.70

A. One or more physical complaints, e.g. fatigue, loss of appetite, gastrointestinal or urinary complaints.

B. Either (1) or (2):

 (1) appropriate evaluation uncovers no organic pathology or pathophysiologic mechanism (e.g. a physical disorder or the effects of injury, medication, drugs, or alcohol) to account for the physical complaints

 (2) when there is related organic pathology, the physical complaints or resulting social or occupational impairment is grossly in excess of what would be expected from the physical findings.

C. Duration of the disturbance of at least six months.

D. Occurrence not exclusively during the course of another Somatoform Disorder, a Sexual Dysfunction, a Mood Disorder, an Anxiety Disorder, a Sleep Disorder, or a psychotic disorder.

Somatoform Disorder Not Otherwise Specified 300.70

Disorders with somatoform symptoms that do not meet the criteria for any specific Somatoform Disorder or Adjustment Disorder with Physical Complaints.

 Examples:

 (1) an illness involving nonpsychotic hypochondriacal symptoms of less than six months' duration

 (2) an illness involving non-stress-related physical complaints of less than six months' duration.

Table 2.3 Proposed classification of psychiatric factors contributing to chronic pain in the International Classification of Diseases, 10th edition

Somatoform disorders

Somatoform pain disorder
Atypical somatoform pain disorder
Multiple somatization disorder
Atypical somatization disorder
Hypochondriacal neurosis

Psychiatric disorders associated with physical conditions

Muscle tension

The criteria for diagnosis of these conditions are very similar to those of DSM-III-R (*see* Table 2.2).

Schema to aid classification of emotional factors

The following questions need to be answered to enable accurate classification:

1 Has there ever been any definite evidence of tissue damage to account for the pain experienced?

The majority of patients with chronic pain have sustained an injury. Acute pain is closely associated with extent of tissue damage but the context in which this occurs may affect the later exhibition of pain. For instance, if the patient believes that when he is first seen by the doctor that there is a serious injury but later investigation fails to confirm any disorder, pain may persist. If pain occurs at the time of a severe physical or emotional trauma this may persist following recovery from the initial injury.

2 Does the patient have a psychiatric illness and, if so, is this as a result of the episode that first caused the pain?

Depression, hypochondriasis, anxiety manifest by muscle tension, somatization disorder and schizophrenia are the main psychiatric diagnoses associated with chronic pain. Depressed patients with pain complaints have similar symptoms to depressed patients who do not have pain. A depressive illness is likely if there has been a measurable change in the quality of the patient's mood accompanied by inability to obtain pleasure from activities that they can still carry out, loss of interest, feelings of hopelessness and weight loss. Hypochondriacal beliefs are common in patients with chronic pain. Those attending chronic pain clinics are usually preoccupied with their pain and when the pain persists despite reassurance from doctors, particularly when they are told that there is nothing organically wrong, it is not unexpected that patients will still hold the belief that they have a disease. However, it is only occasionally that the doctor encounters a patient who is fearful of illness.

Pain arising as a result of anxiety is often associated with muscle tension. Some patients with chronic anxiety contract their muscles to face the unknown threat. The muscles of the neck, head and face are often involved in this exercise and headaches and neck ache are common symptoms. If there is a relationship between the reduction of pain and diminished muscle tension by hypnosis or relaxation the link between signs and symptoms can be established. In practice, close correspondence between muscle tension and pain cannot always be clearly shown even when there are strong grounds for suspecting this.

Somatization disorder arises in late adolescence or early twenties. Patients with this disorder have a history of multiple complaints, often occurring in clusters, for which no sufficient physical cause can be found. It is characteristic of these patients that the locus of symptom changes over time but when complaints are made very many symptoms are exhibited. These individuals have been called 'heartsink' patients and invariably have large medical files.

Pain in schizophrenia is rare and, when it occurs concurrently with this illness, it is usually part of a delusory system. For instance, a patient who complained of numerous painful sites with no evidence of injury and who believed that these were caused by others sticking needles into an effigy of his image would be likely to improve in his pain once his delusory beliefs were controlled.

Finally, although hysterical mechanisms are common in patients with chronic pain it is rare for a patient to have a full hysterical conversion syndrome manifest as chronic pain. In order for a diagnosis of hysteria to be made the symptoms and signs must occur at the time of an emotional conflict and enable the patient to escape or resolve the consequences of this; these same signs must represent the patient's own idea of loss of function in a part of the body and are not due directly to organic pathology. Even if all these three conditions are met the diagnosis of conversion disorders as defined in DSM-III(R) is not permitted if symptoms are confined to pain. Although hysterical pain is a rare occurrence it does occur and this is an important omission in the DSM schedule.

3 Predisposing factors to development of abnormal illness behaviour.

In patients with what used to be called psychogenic pain disorder, now termed somatoform pain disorder in DSM-III(R), there is a higher incidence of certain factors in the personal and past history of patients with this syndrome. Patients with this disorder may show a constellation of factors illustrative of disordered personality development. In some there is a history of taking on responsibilities early on in life, often associated with a 'workaholic' style of life. In these patients a seeming trivial injury may have devastating consequences. These people have high standards and if they do not reach these they may give up. It has been suggested that in these individuals the care and attention they receive when they are ill replaces what they have missed in childhood.

In a separate group of patients there is a history of chronic illness in a close relative, sometimes associated with poor work performance in a manual job. If an injury occurs which enables the patient to apparently legitimately avoid work, persistent pain behaviour may be maintained if other factors also operate.

Conclusion

Few patients with major psychological symptoms associated with their chronic pain can be neatly classified in any one diagnostic symptom. Although depression is common treatment requires more than drugs alone and depression is usually a result of rather than a cause of the pain. There is also the occasional patient with clear manifestations of somatization disorder, hypochondriasis, conversion hysteria or schizophrenia. However, the majority of patients have a mixture of organic pathology, preoccupation with their pain, emotional distress and difficulty in coping and adjusting to their pain. In these cases it is not helpful to classify these patients simply as having psychogenic pain disorder or somatoform pain disorder. Unfortunately under the present DSM-III(R) classification it is not difficult to categorize many patients with these symptoms as suffering from somatoform pain disorder (see Table 2.2). It is more sensible to make a dimensional classification on at least three separate items, psychological distress, muscle tension and extent of hypochondriasis in these patients. In this way, the extent of these factors can be assessed for each patient so that the relative manifestations of each of these attributes are known. This has important prognostic and treatment implications. Patients with significant depression may be appropriately treated with drugs or cognitive therapy, those with muscle tension may benefit from relaxation or hypnosis whereas those with hypochondriacal beliefs may respond to cognitive approaches. Classification along different axes is permitted in a number of classifications, including DSM-III(R), for measures such as personality, social factors and medical conditions. A similar classificatory scheme, perhaps largely based on IASP definitions, would be an advance.

Bibliography

American Psychiatric Association (1987) *Diagnostic and Statistical Manual of Mental Disorders*, 3rd edn (Revised). Washington DC, APA

International Association for the Study of Pain (1986) Classification of chronic pain: descriptions of chronic pain syndromes and definitions of pain terms. *Pain* (Suppl. 3) pp.S5 46–48

World Health Organisation (1990) *International Classification of Diseases*, 10th edn. Draft of Clinical Descriptions and Diagnostic Guidelines. WHO, Geneva

3

Psychological dimensions of chronic pain

P. T. James

In this chapter routine psychology is applied in such a way as to help understand the wide range of individual and unique problems arising from chronic pain. In fact the reader could usefully apply the text to other chronic conditions where there is a noxious sensation, such as tinnitus or itchiness, for the psychological principles are essentially the same. By the end of the chapter, thirty dimensions will be listed which can be used to understand the psychology of pain regardless of the pain site or apparent aetiology.

In contrast to medical models the psychological approach avoids assigning people to discrete categories or diagnosable conditions. Although arguably more difficult at first, the aim is to describe where people are on a continuum or dimension. In Figure 3.1 it can be seen that in the example provided, pain tolerance, different people will have varying levels of pain tolerance. Although the two extremes are of most obvious interest clinically, it is clear that every individual can be allocated a position somewhere on the dimension. The next step is to have a list of such dimensions that actually matter, that is they

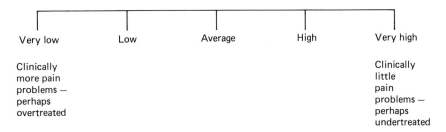

Figure 3.1 *Individual differences in pain tolerance.*

address the problems faced by clinicians and patients alike. This approach is known as the 'multidimensional' model of pain, it is thoroughly described (Karoly and Jensen, 1987), and has clinical utility in guiding practice.

Chronic pain can be split into five broad but distinct dimensions. Firstly, people have a subjective experience which they describe as a *pain sensation*. Secondly, they engage in many thoughts about the pain and its meaning for them; this is known as *pain evaluation*. Thirdly, in association with the sensation and thinking there will necessarily be an emotional experience, or feeling, this being the *pain affect or mood*. Fourthly, the individual in pain will be doing or saying something such as complaining, taking medication or perhaps resting. Not surprisingly, this is known as *pain behaviour*. Finally, the individual's behaviour has an influence or *social impact* on the behaviour and emotions of those connected to them, for example, family, neighbours, employers, doctors and the like.

These five dimensions of pain provide a practical way of grouping together into a hierarchical model the many psychological dimensions which influence pain (summarized later in Table 3.2). This model redefines the question 'What amount of pain?', into the more sophisticated one 'How much of each broad dimension of pain?' As can be seen from later discussions, these dimensions relate closely to each other but it is useful to assess each dimension independently. But the most important fact to remember is that the assessment of a patient's pain is based directly on their pain behaviour and not on the pain sensation. Pain behaviour is influenced not only by pain sensation, the traditional view, but also by the interpretation of the pain experience (pain evaluation) and by mood and the life circumstances. In acute pain there is usually insufficient time for these psychological dimensions to distort the pain experience before the problem is resolved, and so verbal reports of pain behaviour and pain sensation are usually compatible. In chronic pain any clinical assessment must take into account all dimensions for there will be considerable dysynchrony between them.

To illustrate this approach in Figure 3.2, three individuals are depicted. Although they all have the same organic aetiology, one is very emotional (A), one is preoccupied with the meaning of the pain (B), and one is disabled and behaves as excessively sick (C).

Successful interventions will result in an individual who will probably still experience pain sensation but who is minimally disabled in physical and social activities, has minimal emotional distress or affect, and who is not preoccupied mentally by concerns associated with the pain. In the literature this would be described as successful adjustment, and the various approaches people use to deal effectively with their chronic incapacity and painful conditions would be known as coping strategies. The passing from acute pain to chronic pain,

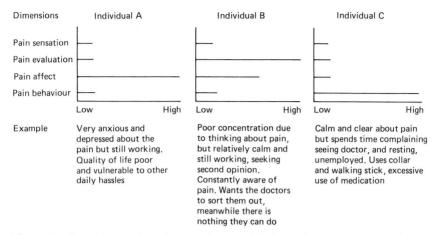

Figure 3.2 *Examples to show the contribution of different dimensions in contributing to pain complaint.*

and then to successful adjustment must be seen as an ongoing process. The health care worker will be assessing at what stage patients are in this process, especially to see if they are stuck before reaching an acceptable adjustment. Quality of life has become the focus, cure has been systematically sought but then abandoned as unrealistic.

Pain sensation

As detailed in Chapter 1 the gate control model of pain (Melzack and Wall, 1982) shows how messages of pain, nerve impulses passing to the pain centre in the brain, can be modified by muscle tension and mood. There are two points to emphasize from this useful model shown and extended in Figure 3.3.

Firstly, this is a real effect on the intensity of pain sensation, it is not the mind playing tricks. This is an important point to make to patients as they will usually want physical and tangible evidence before giving psychological dimensions any credibility. Secondly, mood and muscle tension, regardless of the origin or cause of peripheral pain, will for most pain patients have only a modest effect on pain levels. The effect of physical movement or pressure on pain is usually much greater in comparison with the effect of muscle tension or mood. However, individuals will vary in the degree to which the 'gates' open and close, and for many the difference is enough to make a significant clinical difference.

People differ in their pain threshold, i.e. the amount of physical stimulus to the nerve endings before a sensation of pain is noticed. This is one aspect of pain proneness, i.e. subjects describe severe pain sensation to both current and past events. In such cases the health services tend to overreact. There is some evidence that, broadly

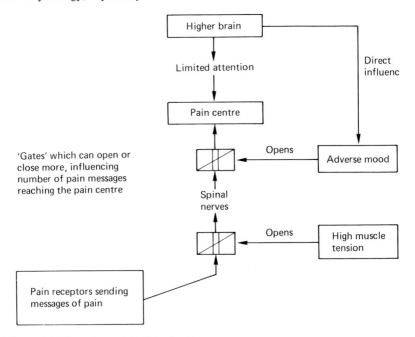

Figure 3.3 *Gate Control Model of pain.*

speaking, extroverted rather than introverted personalities have a lower pain threshold (Bond, 1973). However, a history must be taken, or observation made of reactions to procedures, e.g. tourniquet (*see* Chapter 1), to see what pain threshold each individual has.

In Figure 3.4 reference is made to attention—the capacity humans have to consciously notice certain stimuli from a vast array of internal sensations and external noises, smells and images. Attentional capacity is very limited and so there is a large amount of information processed in the background without the individual becoming consciously aware of it. In chronic pain the problem is reduced if little *pain attention* is given despite messages of pain still being recorded by the pain centre. This is difficult for people who have a tendency or bias to notice internal sensations (Pennebaker, 1982). The greater the bias because of previous illness, degree of introspection or family attentiveness, then the more they will notice a large variety of bodily sensations, including pain. Another dimension is the amount of interesting or novel external stimuli available to an individual with which to distract their attention away from pain; these commonly change after major life events such as death of spouse or with unemployment. The skill an individual has in switching deliberately the attention to non-pain mental events can verbally distract attention from pain; for example, other bodily sensations, environmental sounds, smells and images, thinking and imagery or fantasy. This is known as cognitive displacement (*see* Chapter 11).

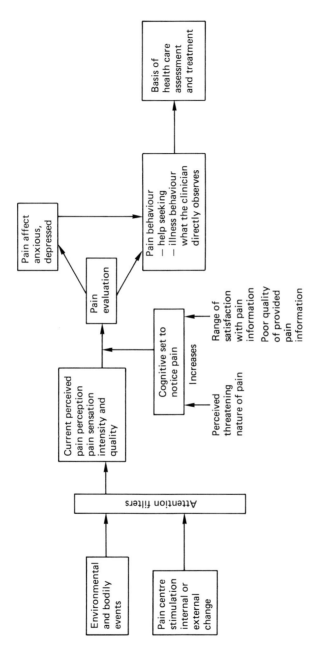

Figure 3.4 *Model showing the interrelationship between pain evaluation, pain sensation, and pain behaviour.*

Once noticed the pain sensation will vary in intensity, which can be roughly estimated by words (none, mild, moderate, severe, and very severe) or by assigning a number (0–10; 10 being pain that could not be more severe). The sensation of pain varies in quality or type, for example, it can be throbbing, dull, piercing or pulling. Such evaluative dimensions will influence the way people interpret their pain. Finally, the pain intensity and quality combine over time to give a noxious experience which may no longer be endured. In experimental studies of pain this occurs when subjects ask that the electrical shocks, or blood tourniquet on the arm, be stopped. In clinical subjects it is more the level of pain which they can cope with. A patient may be experiencing a typical level of pain at six out of ten and want this to be reduced to no pain. The clinician asks: 'Let us assume that the pain cannot be taken away but can be reduced a little, what level of pain can you manage; or get by with?' A reply of five would lead to more optimism about adjustment that an estimate of two. People differ greatly in their pain tolerance level, and this does seem to be influenced by their culture, parental approaches to pain, and their personality. There is ample evidence that pain tolerance levels can be modified.

One final cautionary note is what is actually meant by pain sensation levels in the clinical setting. A reduction in pain sensation intensity, and an increase in the pain threshold or pain tolerance may seem obviously desirable. However, just as important clinically is the time spent with attention 'on' or 'off' the pain sensation. Time spent off an otherwise unchanging pain sensation could constitute a change in pain level. This is a difficult dimension to measure for asking whether they were 'off their pain' obviously puts people back to being 'on' their pain! Unwittingly, many well-meaning families, friends or health care workers are switching people 'on' to their pain in this way. Similarly, asking patients to keep a pain diary can exaggerate the pain normally experienced.

The lower the pain threshold and tolerance, the greater the attentiveness to pain without available distractors, and the more mood disturbance and muscle tension, then the more likely it is that an adequate organic explanation will be unforthcoming, and thus the more resistant to treatment. At its most extreme such an individual predisposition may lead one to suppose that normal neuronal firing in pain pathways can be perceived as pain related illness. This could be called psychogenic pain (*see* Chapter 2).

Pain evaluation

Constantly throughout our wakeful lives we are either attending to and interpreting our environment, or engaging in self-dialogue. We have an excellent system for remembering not only what has happened to us, but also what we see or hear has happened to other people. We have an innate desire to understand events so that we can determine whether we are under threat, and so that we have control. All these cognitive processes have a very powerful effect on how we react to our circumstances. When experiencing chronic pain these cognitive processes will be trying to evaluate the cause, the management and the impact for them of the pain. However, such thinking does not follow the laws of logical science, rather they misunderstand, distort, and selectively remember, to produce a *pain evaluation* unique to them. This is often erroneous on the basis of the perceived sensations (quality and intensity). An individual builds a model in their own head as to what the pain means, i.e. an advancing cancer, pulled muscle, or worn joint. This personal model as to what the pain is, is known as 'illness representation' (Leventhal, Nerenz and Straus, 1980). It will then determine what patients want from the health care services, i.e. more medical investigations, or a cure, and obviously these expectations may go unmet. As we shall see later this illness representation also greatly influences a person's emotional reactions.

To summarize, there is much value in trying to suspend our own professional pain evaluation models and enter into the patient's own perspective. Although it is time consuming the model shown in Figure 3.4 and expanded upon below, demonstrates how this will be greatly influencing the way people describe and react to their condition. From the psychological perspective it is the most central and crucial dimension.

An individual needs information from the health care system, and from informed family or relatives, upon which to base their pain evaluation. Unfortunately all too often the information from the health system is insufficient in amount or clarity. This can arise from clinic time pressure, technical terminology, inconclusive medical investigations, multiple clinical consultations providing different and uncoordinated information, and memory or comprehensive limitations of the patient. Even if the health system has carefully raised the standard of *pain information* to a high level (*see* Chapter 13), problems can still arise. The objective account provided may clash with the individual's own illness representation, or may fall short of the individual's own expectations. When this happens a poor level of *pain information satisfaction* can make the individuals search for more information by second opinions, or make them more dependent upon less reliable lay interpretations.

An individual then uses the available information, which is often patchy and erroneous, to assess the perceived threat that their pain poses to their welfare. Is it life threatening, does it mean another operation, is there an uncertain prognosis? The *pain threat* dimension is usually not overtly expressed by patients, rather the doubt remains in their minds lest they should sound neurotic or silly. In Figure 3.4 the model shows how both low levels of *pain information satisfaction* and high levels of *pain threat* will result in more pain being noticed rather than ignored even though pain sensation levels might be low. This can be described as a *pain cognitive set*. Although with higher levels of pain, the noxious sensation is more likely to 'demand' attention automatically, as the levels of pain intensity decrease the more the pain can be ignored for long periods provided there is a low pain cognitive set.

Pain is usually seen as an acute condition signalling a temporary problem which can be successfully attended to. The medical model of care makes a diagnosis of the problem, and with the expectations that a treatment will be offered by the medical specialist, the patient has to just comply with the treatment regime and all will be well. Unfortunately for many individuals chronic pain remains a condition for which there is no medical cure. Their expectations have to go through a transition from 'an acute problem' to a 'chronic condition'. The transition can be slowed by multiple investigations and medical treatment which all offer the hope of cure. The transition is helped by the passage of time, although it is not uncommon to witness an expectation of cure after ten years of pain. It might be said that given the extraordinary rate of medical advances, it is hard to believe there is nothing that can be done for pain.

There are important consequences stemming from the degree to which there is an expectation of no cure, i.e. *chronic pain acceptance*. Firstly, this will greatly influence the satisfaction and hence compliance with palliative rather than curative medical procedures. Secondly, it will also help determine the amount of health-seeking behaviour, including multiple agency consultations and the seeking of second opinions. Finally, it will be important in predetermining how active an individual is in developing their own way of coping.

Acute pain tends to be associated with a passive role for the patient. In chronic pain the person has to take on an active role in their own pain management because the health service does not have all the answers. This belief in one's own control of pain is known as the *pain locus of control*. In clinical settings the successful passage from a passive (external) to an active (internal) role has been referred to as 'reconceptualization'. Psychologists encourage most individuals to develop an 'internal' sense of control rather than attributing pain control to factors 'external' to them. A crucial distinction here is between the belief that one can significantly control the pain sensation *per se*, or that one can reduce the adverse aspects of chronic pain. The former belief will usually be less realistic and lead to disillusionment, the latter will tend to lead to adaptive behaviour.

Finally, when individuals make the transition to chronic pain acceptance they will weigh up in their minds how much they will have lost. For example, physical disability may cause the loss of jobs with associated loss of income and self-esteem, loss of recreational activities, formerly a source of pleasure, loss of body image, and loss of valued role in the family or neighbourhood. The important dimension here is perceived, rather than actual, *loss from pain*. It is a constellation of changes which we must consider for individuals by understanding what was important to them, and how they currently see their future. For some severely disabled patients the perceived loss is minimal, whereas minor disability for others, perhaps a professional footballer or houseproud person, may be perceived as a major loss. The greater the perceived loss from the pain the more an individual is thrown into a bereavement reaction with all the associated negative emotional, somatic and cognitive consequences. This is discussed in more detail in the next section on pain affect.

For the time being we must recognize that this bereavement process leads eventually to a time when the person *accepts the loss from pain*, though this may be very difficult and be resisted for some time. This dimension has profound implications for clinical management because unwittingly the health system can prolong this unpleasant bereavement process by giving an unrealistic hope of avoiding loss. This 'reassurance' may seem to have short-term benefits but in the long term it is merely putting off what is half acknowledged. Yet at the same time we do not want to encourage people to accept a level of loss which they have over-estimated, as this would lead to excessive disability.

Pain affect

Pain affect directly influences pain perception as described by the gate control model discussed earlier. Similarly in anxiety or stress there is an increase in muscle tension; this can directly cause pain in some conditions where muscles are involved. A depressed affect will lead people to think more negatively about their pain loss and treatment outcome. In successful adjustment the person does not experience extremes of anxiety or depression, for this obviously has an adverse effect on the quality of life. For these reasons we must have a basic understanding of emotions both to ensure that these are not excessively magnifying the pain problem, and to provide services that facilitate emotional adjustment. Our discussion must consider premorbid emotionality, and non-pain problems causing background emotional distress, because these factors accumulate to influence pain affect (Figure 3.5). It is all too easy for the clinician and patient to attribute the emotional distress to either the pain *or* to life events, whereas in fact there will inevitably be an interaction of problems.

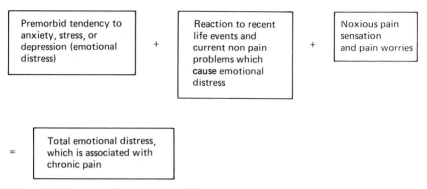

Figure 3.5 *Factors influencing pain affect.*

Anxiety and stress

Let us first consider anxiety and stress. Both describe a state of the individual where there is increased bodily activation, particularly that associated with the sympathetic nervous system. The greater this bodily activation the greater the anxiety or stress. The more prolonged the bodily activation and the less opportunity to recover, then the more chronically anxious and the more widespread the stress-related problems become. This includes difficulty in sleeping, irritability, a variety of somatic sensations such as palpitations, muscle aches and headaches, and possibly a tendency towards panic attacks. Figure 3.6 illustrates the primacy of thoughts in dictating whether or not a physical reaction occurs, which is then perceived as either stress or anxiety.

In chronic pain many of these anxiety- or stress-inducing thoughts may be pain related, but other daily hassles and life events will produce stress-producing thoughts. It can be seen that pain sensation itself tends to automatically cause a physical reaction; it is like a universal stressor, and so causes greater emotionality. Unfortunately those with a premorbid tendency to strong emotions will find the pain pushes them to unacceptable emotional levels in the absence of other stressors. The model also indicates that life stressors can themselves produce pain by resulting in excessive physical stimulation in vulnerable organs. Head pain or 'irritable bowel' pain are examples. This might help explain the initial pain onset for some patients. More usually this helps explain how anxiety or stress can exacerbate an existing pain. Hence a vicious circle is established: pain and perceived threat/demand cause anxiety/stress; anxiety and stress cause more pain and perceived threat/demand. These dimensions accumulate to increase the emotional distress which is attached to the pain phenomenology. The clinical implications of anxiety or stress are discussed in Chapters 10 and 11.

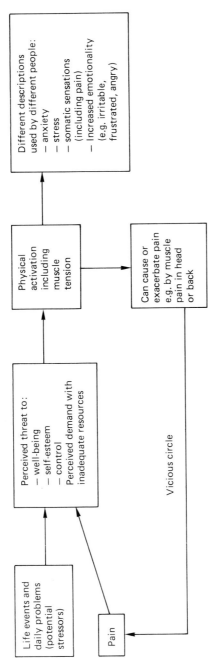

Figure 3.6 *Psychological model of anxiety or stress.*

Unhappiness, hopelessness, helplessness and depression

In a chronic pain population there is a high prevalence of significant unhappiness, clinical depression, and suicidal ideas. As with anxiety or stress these are often alien and frightening experiences, which for some may suggest that they are 'weak and cracking up'. To others it is confirmation that, as an adequate organic basis to their pain has not been found, the hospital's assertions that their problem is functional may be well-founded. It is also very easy to take a pathological view of depression and treat with antidepressants. In this section the reader should be able to see that a depressed and hopeless/helpless mood associated with chronic pain is readily understandable, and that there are alternatives to medical treatment based on psychological principles (see Chapter 11).

The starting point is to recognize the primacy of thoughts in determining mood (Beck, 1976). In Figure 3.7 it can be seen that if for whatever reason a person starts to think negatively about their own worth (self-esteem), thinks life currently has little to offer them, or can see little future for themselves, then they become depressed. It is then that energy, appetite, sleep, concentration and libido become adversely affected. Such physical symptoms associated with mood disturbance can then be attributed to their physical condition and hence magnify the perceived gravity of their illness.

The next step in understanding depressive affect is to consider the impact of chronic pain for the individuals. Does it take away activities or roles which were an important source of self-esteem? Does the idea of being partially disabled seem particularly hurtful to their body image? Has the pain taken away important sources of enjoyment or relaxation? Have ambitions or ideas about the future been severely threatened by their view of their pain? Remember it is not the reality of the situation, but the individual's own perceptions which will determine the depressed mood. Finally, people differ in their premorbid vulnerability to depression because of their tendency to think negatively, and also other life events may induce negative thinking (see Figure 3.5). Consequently the clinician will try to distinguish between these three dimenions (*trait depressive thinking, life event induced thinking*, and *pain-induced depressive thinking*), for the clinical implications are quite different (see Chapter 11).

There are two special variants of depression which are worth expanding upon, one is learned helplessness and the second is loss and bereavement. When individuals want something very much (to be pain free or to increase their behavioural activity), believe they should be able to do something, and yet despite their every effort repeatedly do not succeed, then they learn that they are helpless to effect change. Such learned helplessness is marked by a sense of helplessness and inactivity, this being similar to depression. They can

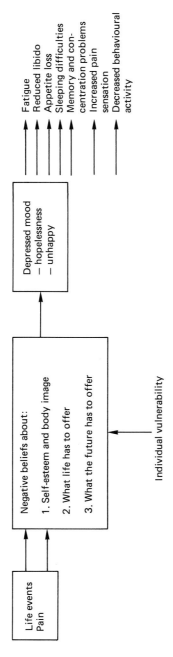

Figure 3.7 *Model showing how depressed mood can follow from chronic pain.*

remain in this passive state not bothering to try and move. The clinical implications of this *learned helplessness dimension* are explored in Chapter 11. The second variant of depression results from perceived loss (*see* pain evaluation dimensions), the pain affect then is seen as part of an unavoidable bereavement reaction. There will be a period of grieving for what things were like, similar to that resulting from the loss of someone close. Typically there are a variety of strong emotions including anger (probably at the health service), frustration, and depression which it would seem need expressing openly to facilitate the bereavement process (Worden, 1991). In the clinic this will probably be accompanied by an apparent worsening of their pain problem (*see* Figure 3.3).

Pain behaviour

It is by assessing pain behaviour that the clinician makes a diagnosis and offers treatment. Furthermore the extent of pain behaviour has an enormous influence on the quality of life for both individuals and their family. However, pain behaviour is influenced by a range of factors other than pain sensation (*see* Figure 3.4). From a clinical point of view we are particularly interested in why it is that some individuals engage in excessive pain reporting and health care seeking behaviour compared with others. They run the serious risk of becoming overtreated, or causing a negative reaction towards them from health care staff. These individuals are excessively disabled by their pain and this leads to a poorer quality of life because of restrictions they impose on their activities.

There are different types of pain behaviour, although they are all subject to the same basic psychological laws. A list of pain behaviours is given in Table 3.1 which can be seen as making up the behavioural repertoire, yet each can be disproportionately high or low in frequency. Some of the associated clinical problems are noted to illustrate the range of 'behavioural' problems that can present with chronic pain.

Pain sensation and pain affect have a motivating property; people will engage in behaviour where the desired outcome is to alleviate the noxious experiences. Consequently the greater the pain sensation and pain affect, then generally the more pain behaviour there will be. What the subjects actually do will depend upon their pain evaluation, that is their beliefs about cause and management. Some of this pain behaviour will be consciously determined, others will be subconscious. For example, conscious and persistent *help-seeking behaviour* may stem from a pain evaluation which leads to expectations that more can still be done. Perhaps unconsciously subjects may be exaggerating their *pain-reporting behaviour* on the principle that you get a service if you make a nuisance of yourself. Alternatively, a person may be

Table 3.1 The pain behavioural repertoire showing possible behavioural problems

Type of pain behaviour	Examples	Associated problems	
		In excess	If deficient
Pain reporting	Verbal ratings non-vocal grimaces, posture	Over-invasive therapies, e.g. surgery	Under-use of available help
Help seeking	Multiple clinic visits	Negative reaction from health care—confusion from different disciplines	Under-use of available help
Sick	As above, limps, bed rest	People expect less, become disabled	Exposure to further injury
Compliance	Medication, use of TNS	Over-dependent and passive, not experimenting with own coping strategies	Cannot benefit from structured help
Avoidance	Pain behaviour to stop doing something else which is unpleasant or difficult, e.g. avoid job responsibility	Unnecessarily disabled and restricted	Exposure to high levels of pain or stress
Well (incompatible with pain behaviour)	Living life as normally as possible, e.g. working hobbies	Push themselves too far, perhaps not adjusted, cause further injury	No distraction from pain, nothing to enjoy, or look forward to (depressogenic)

motivated to try an excessive range of tactics, including medications and physical aids, because logically from their point of view it makes sense to try these illness behaviours. Yet again, they might be applying routinely a technique such as transcutaneous electrical nerve stimulation three times a day for a year but without effect, because they believe that they should follow the doctor's and nurse's instructions (pain compliance). In all these examples, the pain behaviour would be understandable if the individual's pain evaluation had been understood.

A completely different explanation of how pain behaviours can arise is through the shaping of behaviour by reinforcement and punishment. Without consciously being aware, our behaviour is shaped up by what happens immediately afterwards. This is known as operant conditioning. If the outcome is a good one (reinforcement), that behaviour becomes more intense and frequent, the opposite happens when the outcome is unpleasant (punishment). So if pain behaviour is followed by something we need or want such as attention from our spouse or doctor, payments, or control over a relative, then that pain behaviour is unconsciously increased. The pain sensation in these examples remains unchanged. Similarly every time pain behaviour, such as taking medication, is reinforced by pain reduction, that pain behaviour is strengthened until it becomes disproportionate to the pain sensation. Again this occurs automatically without the subject being aware of it.

Rest is also reinforced by pain reduction until this becomes a major illness behaviour. Unfortunately too much leads to contraction of fibres in inactive muscles. This in turn produces secondary pain on subsequent use, and so well behaviour becomes punished. Such pain is often attributed incorrectly to the original damage and so rest continues. This pattern is particularly common, and a therapeutic strategy to reverse this trend can theoretically be easily worked out (*see* Chapters 9 and 11). Additional reinforcers are given specifically following appropriate activity which leads to muscle fibres lengthening; this offsets the punishment aspect of increased pain. In all these examples the pain behaviour will gradually change frequency and intensity as long as the reinforcement or punishment alters, e.g. spouse no longer gives attention.

Perhaps of more importance because of its persistent qualities is avoidance behaviour. This occurs when an individual routinely and almost superstitiously behaves in a way to avoid doing something that is unconsciously or consciously judged to be distressing. In chronic pain, well behaviour is avoided because of anticipated pain, even though subsequent pain may not be experienced. Associated features include the holding of certain body postures thought initially to protect the individual from pain. Unfortunately this body posture may itself produce muscle pain. A more subtle encouragement of pain behaviour occurs when the pain stops an individual doing something unrelated to pain that has been found unpleasant or stressful, e.g. unsatisfactory job or unwanted sexual demands. This is also avoidance behaviour, but the advantage is secondary to pain. Again this type of behaviour can be very resistant to change.

Another interesting application of operant conditioning is to well behaviour, e.g. vocational and recreational activities. We engage in these because they are rewarding; if they were to stop being rewarding, then gradually these activities would reduce in frequency according to behavioural principles, i.e. unrewarded behaviour gradually diminishes. When either the pain is in a bad phase, or the pain is being magnified by pain effect and/or pain evaluation styles, then *well behaviour* may stop because of the temporarily increased pain which reduces the enjoyment. When the period of worsened pain passes, the well behaviour does not necessarily reappear even though in these new circumstances it would be rewarding. The individual's well behaviour repertoire could then be permanently restricted, especially when there is no encouragement from family or friends to renew former pastimes.

Social context

When an individual experiences pain he or she will have an influence on their family and friends, for example, the immediate family may also suffer a loss of income and freedom. There may be a change of role in the family, for example, from dominant to submissive. The family may experience distress vicariously. Families can themselves become entrenched in the illness behaviour, for example, managing or encouraging compliance. The *family impact* of pain is not only relevant because of the relatives' quality of life, but also because the families' reaction will in turn influence the pain sufferer. For example, marital satisfaction often suffers in 30% of chronic pain patients, and this in turn can be a stressor which exacerbates pain. Particularly important is the family pain evaluation because the family is often more influential than the health care providers in shaping up the patient's pain evaluation; also the family could be inadvertently reinforcing the pain behaviour. Perhaps to have a spouse sick with pain has advantages. The family may be discouraging *well behaviour* thinking that they are appropriately protecting their loved ones from further pain. In chronic pain it is worthwhile considering the individual within their family context. This is quite unusual in routine medical practice. *See* Chapters 9 and 11 for more details.

It is not only the family but also the health care system which both influences, and reacts, to patients. For example, medical science and its advances leads to expectations that a successful diagnosis or cure can be reached. Such attitudes obviously shape patients' expectations, but also those of health workers. The medical model also tends to view the patient as uninformed, yet in chronic pain management the healthcare professional wishes to encourage the patient to develop a set of coping strategies. The health care system also has a tendency to become intolerant with pain presentation when no organic pathology can be found. To explain this the terms psychogenic or functional may be used with all its ambiguous connotations. Staff tend to react negatively to such patients, perhaps projecting their own frustration. Beyond the health care system our society may give financial incentives for people to stay sick, and doctors may collude, thinking this from the patient's perspective to be the best option. A culture may even reward sick or illness behaviour with 'prevailing attitudes' such as 'isn't he doing well despite his disability'. The social dimension of

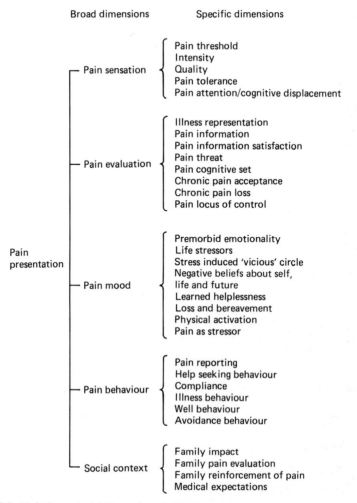

Figure 3.8 *Multidimensional hierarchy of chronic pain.*

chronic pain gives a better insight into the way a patient thinks about and behaves with their pain. Chapter 6 illustrates this social-cultural dimension with different compensation systems in different countries.

Summary

In this chapter a large number of psychological dimensions have been covered, shown hierarchically in Figure 3.8. When added together they give us a comprehensive way of describing and understanding each person who is asking for help. No apologies are given for the fact that there are a lot of different problems that can occur; this is the real world clinically.

To start with we must first choose the most obvious problematic dimensions, perhaps starting with pain behaviour, and devise assessment questionnaires or structured clinical interviews to assess them. But then as we become more psychologically sophisticated we can become sensitive to a wider range of dimensions. As a result we will at the very least be able to empathise more fully with the patient and the family, an important therapeutic process detailed later (Chapter 11), regardless of the pain aetiology. The chapter will have shown that there is a 'functional overlay' to some degree in all individuals who present with chronic pain. Trying to argue whether this is of sufficient magnitude to call it 'psychogenic overlay' does seem rather futile, especially as the term is associated with prejudice in both staff and patients.

An alternative is to screen the overall pain syndrome, including sensation, affect, evaluation, behaviour and social context to see whether there are any disproportionate or excessive dimensions. Unfortunately all too often health staff, families, and individuals with pain fail to understand the psychological complexity. This results in a restricted range of therapeutic options. Employing the multi-dimensional model to pain gives rise to many new ways of helping patients and families improve their quality of life.

Bibliography

Beck, A. T. (1976) *Cognitive Therapy and the Emotional Disorders.* International Universities Press, New York

Bond, M. (1973) Personality studies in patients with pain secondary to organic disease. *Journal of Psychosomatic Research*, **17**, 257–263

Karoly, P. and Jensen, M. P. (1987) *Multimethod Assessment of Chronic Pain.* Pergamon Press, Oxford

Leventhal, H., Meyer, D. and Nerenz, D. (1980) The common sense representation of illness danger. In *Contributions to Medical Psychology* (ed. S. Rachman), Pergamon Press, Oxford

Leventhal, H., Nerenz D. and Straus, A. (1980) Self-regulation and the mechanisms for symptom appraisal. In *Psychosocial Epidemiology* (ed. Mechanic, D.), Neal Watson, New York, pp. 353–389.

Melzack, R. and Wall, P. (1982) *The Challenge of Pain.* Penguin Books, Harmondsworth

Pennebaker, J. W. (1982) *The Psychology of Physical Symptoms.* Springer-Verlag, New York

Sternbach, R. A. (1986) *The Psychology of Pain.* Raven Press, New York

Worden, J. W. (1991) *Grief Counselling and Grief Therapy.* Routledge, London

4

Chronic pain problems and psychiatry

H. Merskey and P. Chandarana

The relationship between pain and psychological factors has been described in full in earlier chapters. It is clear that states of anxiety and some other psychological conditions may promote or induce pain. It is also evident that changes in the emotional state may relieve, reduce or abolish pain. Indeed pain always has to be thought of as a psychological phenomenon. It is not the actual events in nerve fibres or receptor endings but a subjective experience in the mind of an individual—whoever may be suffering from it. It is for these reasons that the International Association for the Study of Pain adopted the following definition: 'An unpleasant sensory and emotional experience associated with actual or potential tissue damage, or described in terms of such damage' (IASP, 1979).

One of the most important reasons for this definition is to permit the understanding that psychological illness may be a cause of pain which is just as valid as any physical illness promoting pain. Shortly, we will review the psychiatric states that produce pain, themselves. By this we mean states of mind or psychological illness in which the individual develops the experience of pain just defined above, in some part of the body. Later in this chapter, we also look at the emotional changes which may be produced by chronic physical illness causing pain. The psychiatric factors contributing to chronic pain are listed in Table 4.1.

Our discussion here deals essentially with chronic pain. With respect both to acute pain and chronic pain, however, we can summarize one important aspect of pain by recognizing that moderate arousal increases pain whilst high arousal may abolish it. Anxious individuals generally feel more pain from a given stimulus than those who are relaxed and tranquil. In circumstances of the highest arousal, e.g. battle and some vigorous sports, pain may be less prominent or even absent when it would normally be anticipated to be present. That is

Table 4.1 Psychiatric factors involved in chronic pain

Cause or mental mechanisms	Significance in patients with chronic pain
Anxiety	Increased anxiety associated with increased pain. Pain may be reduced or even absent under conditions of very high anxiety. May play a significant part if anxiety is associated with muscle tension
Depression	Commonest psychiatric symptom in patients with chronic pain. Endogenous depression found at most in 10–15% of all cases. Depression is usually a result of the pain. Irritability common
Hysteria	Difficult to evaluate as no loss of function with hysterical pain as opposed to conversion disorders. Not uncommon but often no more than unconscious increase in existing symptoms for a variety of motives. Isolated cases where pain provides a solution for an unconscious conflict
Hypochondriasis	The element of disease conviction is very common particularly in patients with no demonstrable evidence of physical illness Actual fear about disease is not uncommon. The important mechanism is misinterpretation of mild body sensations

Patients with Briquet syndrome or somatization disorder display a combination of hypochondriacal and hysterical symptoms and seek medical help for a wide variety of personal problems

Drug dependence	Commoner in patients given opiates. More likely in patients with personality disorder; particularly passive-dependent personalities
Psychosis	Rare but definite cases of pain can arise in schizophrenia and psychotic depression; occasionally in monosymptomatic hypochondriacal psychosis

These items are given in order of approximate frequency, not in order of their significance in directly causing pain.

not the whole explanation for the absence of pain. A high proportion of patients in a hospital emergency department, amounting to approximately one-third, was observed by Melzack, Wall and Ty (1982) not to have pain at the time of examination even though it might well have been anticipated from the nature of the injuries. Some of that might have been due to shock, initially, more than to high arousal. Also some pain from injuries takes time to evolve, e.g. that from a cervical hyperextension injury may not appear for hours or days. In any event the absence of pain following injury may be due to high arousal but is not always attributable to that cause. Nevertheless the curvilinear relationship which has been indicated is important. Very low and very high arousal both seem to be related to an absence of pain. Intermediate arousal and anxiety above the average level usually result in increased pain or pain where it would not otherwise be present, at least in clinical practice.

Monism of experience and dualism of aetiology

The definition of pain which has been given, treats it as an experience and avoids any implications about current causes. It is recognized that the experience is related to past events linked with trauma. We identify a particular type of experience or group of experiences on the basis of physical injury or changes in the body with which they are recognized as being associated. Nevertheless, these experiences are solely subjective and philosophically are a monistic concept. We see them as a category which is related to the mind and unitary, not dependent upon any physical interactions or causes for their acceptance. It would be a mistake to think of pain or any other aspect of mental activity as something which appears because of an interaction between the body and the mind. That sort of thinking confuses two sets of terms, one dealing with our subjective experience and psychological concepts, the other dealing with our concepts of the physical state of the body, including the brain. This sort of psychophysical parallelism is best avoided in trying to deal with the body/mind relationship. Instead we should look upon the events which we call pain as a set of events which we are describing in psychological terms, the same events being open to description in physical terms if we have enough physical knowledge about the brain. But one is not the other. Each is a different set of terms for an occurrence or set of occurrences.

This separation of psychology and physiology is very convenient and logical with regard to the experience. It is disadvantageous and unnecessary with regard to aetiology. We can recognize that a set of occurrences in one field may have antecedents in both fields. Headache can be as well provoked by a blow as by an emotional conflict. There need be no problem in accepting multiple aetiology, i.e. dualism, and more if we wish, whilst insisting on the monistic nature of pain itself as an experience.

For the philosophical this can be summarized as monism of substance or properties and a dualism of aetiologies. In practice it means not worrying that we accept that the patient's state is a psychological one, pain, although the causes that contribute to this are diverse and often will be of a physical nature.

Psychiatric diagnosis and organic diagnosis

It is common and wrong for psychiatric illness to be diagnosed because of the absence of evidence of physical illness. It is correct that the failure to find a physical cause of sufficient importance should lead the clinician to look at the possibility of a psychiatric cause being relevant. In this situation the practitioner of health care should be ready to conduct psychological or psychiatric evaluation without feeling obliged to make a psychiatric diagnosis. Most psychiatric diagnoses declare themselves quite readily. The patient is aware of significant anxiety, evidence of depression is very obvious, or a well-marked syndrome of hypochondriacal over-emphasis with varied symptoms may be apparent. In such circumstances the supplementary information which is necessary to complete a psychiatric diagnosis, in terms of sufficient features of a syndrome and sufficient reason for it being present, can usually be found. However a proportion of cases exists—varying with the clinic or centre—in which neither adequate physical evidence appears to explain pain, nor a sufficient psychiatric explanation is found. In these circumstances it is important not to accept the view that the condition is psychiatric. It is more appropriate to suspend judgement, re-examine psychologically on another occasion, extend the process of data gathering, in the psychiatric field by interviewing a member of the family, or even seek a little more organic investigation. There can be no absolute position in this matter, only a willingness to review and adjust the interpretation of the clinical data according to what can reasonably be made available.

Perhaps one of the outstanding examples of the problem under consideration exists in the DSM-III(R) criteria for the so-called somatoform pain disorder (American Psychiatric Association, 1987). This category in the DSM-III(R) still, like the corresponding category of psychogenic pain disorder in DSM-III, allows the diagnosis of a psychological condition to be made if there is insufficient evidence of a physical cause and there is apparently proportionate stress to which the condition might be attributed. The consequence of applying this rule to conditions which might have a subtle and insufficiently recognized physical cause was shown by Fishbain et al. (1986) who found that 38% of their patients who had myofascial pain disorder also fulfilled the DSM-III criteria for conversion disorder.

This diagnosis was made because these patients had a symptom, such as sensory abnormalities, that could not readily be explained on the basis of the known pathology of myofascial syndromes. However, there are now good reasons for supposing that non-dermatomal sensory abnormalities have a physiological basis.

It would obviously be a serious matter and a difficult clinical situation to make a diagnosis of conversion disorder (or the pain equivalent, which is normally somatoform pain disorder under DSM-

III(R)), if in fact, the patients have a poorly understood physical problem. This would be a difficulty in one case, never mind 38% of one's practice.

In fact this issue arises repeatedly and the diagnosis of hysteria or so-called psychogenic pain is often made on patients with chronic pain with insufficient justification, at least in the light of modern knowledge. Explanation of this problem requires a little further discussion.

The diagnosis of hysteria is a broad one which can cover a number of phenomena but for the purpose of this discussion can be limited to recognizing whether or not a symptom is a 'conversion disorder'. There are two ways of defining conversion disorder. In both methods one has to say that it corresponds to a patient's idea of a symptom rather than to the necessary physiological and anatomical phenomena which correspond to loss of use or dysfunction. In both instances also there is usually a loss of function but pain may be considered to be a hysterical symptom as well.

In the first method of confirmation the symptom is explained psychodynamically as resolving an unconscious conflict with which the patient is faced. If psychological exploration and evaluation of the circumstances provide enough evidence, this attribution will be justifiable. This method of explanation and confirmation is available for pain if it is a hysterical symptom. It is also available for other types of symptoms such as paralysis or anaesthesia.

The second method of confirmation depends upon physical examination and is not available for pain. It requires a demonstration that the symptoms not only do not correspond to the physical characteristics which are normally anticipated, such as distribution according to a dermatome or set of muscle groups, but also are accompanied by positive action in muscles or positive function in a sensory system which the patient believes he or she has lost. Thus, typically, in neurological examination, it can be demonstrated that the patient is able to do things with muscles which he believes to be paralysed. One of the favourite examples occurs in the case of hysterical paralysis of a leg. Raising the 'well' leg will be accompanied in a hysterical case by use of the hip extensors and knee flexors to press the supposedly paralysed leg down in order to counter-balance the raising of the good limb. This shows that, despite the patient's belief, there is function in particular muscles. This demonstration by means of a 'positive sign' is probably the best form of evidence that a particular symptom is hysterical, other than the recovery of the symptom after psychological exploration and the resolution of conflicts.

Only the technique of psychological exploration is available to confirm a diagnosis of hysterical pain. In the past (Merskey, 1965) hysteria has also been diagnosed for pain when the symptom was found as part of a complex of other somatic symptoms (somewhat comparable to somatization disorder) and this may still be justified if the variety of psychological symptoms is sufficient. Hysterical personality may also be recognized in association with pain whatever its cause. Nevertheless attributing pain in association with a hysterical personality to a conversion symptom will often be unsound.

It is further noteworthy that two of the major signs on physical examination which are often used to promote the diagnosis of hysterical pain are not reliable. Most of the so-called 'soft' signs of hysteria are mimicked by organic disease (Gould et al., 1986). The most notable example of this is so-called giveway weakness. Many patients with pain will voluntarily or involuntarily refuse to undertake movements during physical examination which they know will produce pain, even though the actual capacity to perform the movement is available. This is often called hysterical but in fact is better described as 'pain inhibition'. It cannot be relied upon, as it often is unfortunately, to sustain a diagnosis of pain of psychological origin.

Secondly, there is a physiological basis for regional pain and also for some of the hypoaesthesias and diminutions in sensory sensitivity which are associated with regional pain syndromes. It is well recognized that in the presence of a painful lesion in one part of a limb a diffuse increase in sensitivity and spontaneous pain may be found elsewhere across dermatomal boundaries. This is likely particularly to be the case with the myofascial pain syndrome which is increasingly recognized as a diagnosable entity. In that syndrome only a minority of patients is thought to have evidence of psychiatric illness (Ahles, Yunus and Masi, 1987). Individual nociceptive cells in the dorsal horn will also respond to stimulation from receptor fields which are much wider than a single dermatome. Hence the idea should be abandoned that because a patient complains of a regional pain syndrome it is necessarily hysterical. The plasticity of the nervous system in supporting sensory phenomena or altering them in the presence of chronic pain is a plausible explanation of these clinical phenomena.

The importance of these findings for the health care practitioner is that they undermine the diagnosis of hysteria in many cases of chronic pain to which it has been too readily applied; and it is always best for the psychologist or psychiatrist not to have to cure a supposed psychological illness for which a physical diagnosis and remedy are more appropriate.

The process of selection

If the process of diagnosis has proceeded satisfactorily the significance of a relationship between pain and a psychological condition may still require special consideration. Anyone with a longlasting condition that is mostly not progressive and not fatal has a wide range of choices about whom he will see with respect to his complaint and what he will do about it. Some individuals with phlegmatic characteristics will do little except tolerate the disorder and continue with their normal activities. They may try an over-the-counter preparation from a pharmacy, and on mature consideration decide that it does not help them, or that it gives about the right amount of relief. They may not even go to a doctor at all.

Most people who have an acute condition which they think needs a medical remedy will consult doctors. The difference between the way different symptoms are treated is illuminated by a study from general practice by Banks et al. (1975) who showed that only 3% of all the daily symptoms which individuals experienced were actually reported to their general practitioners. Headache was rarely taken to the general practitioner. Sore throat was often a matter for consultation. We can reasonably assume that the individuals who persist in attending their practitioner because of chronic pain will represent a special sample of all chronic pain patients. Those who go to pain clinics will represent a further sample filtered by the general practitioner. Those who go to many specialists, and particularly to the most distant and least accessible in far countries at famous clinics, will represent the most highly filtered group of all. In fact those in pain clinics have been shown to complain of more severe pain than those not in pain clinics and also to have a number of other characteristics which separate them from pain patients found in the community (Crook and Tunks, 1985).

It is actually very hard to think of any non-fatal disorder which is not liable to have some sampling bias amongst hospital populations. Even if one considers coronary infarction or similar disorders the individuals who do or do not seek treatment will have particular characteristics. Perhaps only cases brought in dead to casualty departments because of some unknown prior disorder, such as a silent aneurysm, will represent a true sample of the general population, unbiased by psychological selection factors.

All this means that the features of chronic pain patients which are important may not be absolute. They deserve attention because the individuals who need treatment have them; but some of them should not be understood as the primary cause of their pain. They may, however, be a major cause of the need for medical attention.

Psychiatric diagnosis in pain patients

If even the patients in general practice are subject to a selection effect, such an effect can only be greater when different study populations are examined from sources varying from psychiatric hospitals to nerve block clinics.

The initial psychiatric work defining the characteristics of one type of chronic pain patients was undertaken mostly in patients attending a university psychiatric department. These studies showed that if patients were examined who had had pain for more than three months, who presented it as a major complaint, who were defined as being thought likely to have psychiatric illness, and who did not have a physical disorder, then a substantial minority of the patients would be found to have depression of one sort or another and the majority would have had neurotic conditions including anxiety and hysterical phenomena. Those hysterical phenomena principally included a past history of possible conversion symptoms or personality problems (Merskey, 1965). They did not specifically define the pain as hysterical in modern terms except on the basis of indirect evidence. In the same locations of clinic and hospital, patients who had pain were also examined by Spear (1967). In his study all pain was counted whether spontaneously reported or not, and whether of short duration or long. The bulk of the pain was then found to be associated with diagnoses of anxiety and depression, with less emphasis on hypochondriasis and hysteria, although these phenomena were still linked somewhat to pain in psychiatric patients.

In most pain clinics it is assumed that the patients are referred primarily, after appropriate diagnosis, for nerve blocks or other procedures aimed at alleviating symptoms of pain from a physical cause. In recent years there has been an increasing tendency to recognize that many patients will need psychological or behavioural management within the pain clinic. Be that as it may the initial assumption must be that pain clinic patients have a high frequency of individuals with somatic causes of pain whatever additional psychological phenomena are to be found. The classic description of pain clinic patients and their varied characteristics was provided by Sternbach (1974). In these cases the emphasis has been substantially on hysterical phenomena, hypochondriacal characteristics and the so-called 'conversion V pattern' of the Minnesota Multiphasic Personality Inventory (MMPI). Reservations have been expressed concerning the application of the MMPI and its interpretation in that context.

A number of authors including Watson (1982), Naliboff, Cohen and Yellen (1983) and Weekes et al. (1983), amongst others, have pointed out that the somatic complaints which may appear with chronic pain for physical reasons are liable to be confused with somatic complaints made in the absence of physical illness. Hence the simple counting of these items in the MMPI distorts their significance. Nevertheless for practical purposes it remains the case that the emphasis on somatic complaints, sometimes disproportionate to the demonstrable physical state, is the commonest clinical pattern in those patients in pain clinics who are thought to have psychological disturbance. Somatization, or in the older language, hysteria and hypochondriasis, is thus relatively more pronounced. It may be no more than a tendency for patients with a physical illness to select themselves by emphasis upon their physical condition as discussed above, or it may go so far as a fundamental hysterical conversion symptom. The latter is hard to prove, however, for the reasons already outlined.

The problems of measuring instruments such as the MMPI, clinical assessment, and the samples of patients to be examined, have been reviewed by Romano and Turner (1985) with particular reference to patients with depression. A widely varying prevalence both of depressive symptoms and of diagnosable depression in pain patients (10–80%) was observed as well as a widely varying prevalence of pain symptoms in patients who were clinically depressed (27–100%).

Discrepancies also result from a failure to distinguish between the presence of various depressive symptoms, e.g. tearfulness, sadness, diminished interest in activities etc. and the presence of a specific affective disorder, particularly diagnosable major depression, according to the DSM-III(R) of the American Psychiatric Association (1987). Tyrer et al. (1989), using the Present State Examination, showed that in a pain clinic series, 21% of the patients had a depressive disorder. These findings seem to fit fairly well with the current experience in pain clinics.

One of us (H.M.) in his personal service for patients with chronic pain undertook an assessment according to DSM-III of 32 patients randomly selected, for the presence of psychiatric illness at any time in the course of their painful illness (Merskey et al., 1987). Nine patients had major affective disorder according to DSM-III, 12 had an atypical affective disorder, 3 had anxiety disorders and one each had conversion symptoms, hypochondriasis and dementia. No psychiatric disorder was found in 5. This is a highly selected sample in which approximately two-thirds had some degree of diagnosable depressive illness at some time. Other sorts of data from the same patients taken on a cross-sectional basis, during screening for psychiatric illness, showed lower rates of actual psychiatric diagnoses.

All pain clinics will contain a number of patients, also with variable frequencies, who have undue somatization problems. They will also all contain some patients who have developed problems with medication, whether that be narcotic medication such as codeine, often in compound tablet form, or the benzodiazepines. Substance abuse and occasional or more frequent alcoholism must therefore be expected. The alcoholism may be symptomatic of depression or a response directly to the pain. It may of course be independent and *sui generis*. There will also be a few, rather rare, cases of schizophenic types of illness, as well as the occasional patient who dwells on a single delusional idea concerning the body, known as monosymptomatic hypochondriacal psychosis. The depression found will often be associated with anxiety. It will most often be a reactive depression in type and less often an endogenous pattern.

In the authors' observations the commonest psychiatric patterns in pain clinics or in personal practice are of depression of mild to moderate severity, secondary to physical illness. Some of the criteria for depression which are often employed cannot be wholly relied upon in this context, including insomnia and fatigue since these symptoms may be provoked either by pain or by medication. However, the patients do commonly show sadness, a loss of ability to concentrate or attend to other matters, impaired energy and a good deal of irritability. The latter is relatively common in painful syndromes and may well be a more marked feature in depression linked with pain than in other sorts of depression. Marital friction is also common in these cases. The patients are misdiagnosed at times as having 'adjustment reactions' and fail to receive appropriate antidepressant therapy.

The second most common psychiatric phenomena will be those related to anxiety. There will be a miscellaneous group of patients as indicated, with substance abuse, perhaps personality disorders, a marked tendency to somatization or hypochondriasis and even, occasionally, clear evidence of a psychodynamic conflict which is producing a conversion symptom. Whereas formerly we used to consider that the hysterical symptoms were the most common features of psychiatric illness in patients with chronic pain, we think that this interpretation should be revised with respect to current practice.*

In all cases, however, the practitioner should recognize the common finding that both physical and psychological factors coexist. This in turn should lead to a comprehensive plan of treatment for the patient.

The effects of pain

The effects of chronic pain in causing emotional change are implied above. In particular we think of irritability as a consequence of chronic pain. Weir Mitchell (1872) described emotional changes in his patients who had suffered from injuries of nerves. In one case he wrote 'from being a man of gay and kindly temper, known in his company as a good natured jester, he became morose and melancholy and complained that reading gave him vertigo, and that his memory of recent events was bad'. Woodforde and Merskey (1972) found evidence that patients with pain due to physical lesions were actually more anxious, more depressed, and more subject to signs of neuroticism than a comparison

---

* Likewise the diagnosis of somatoform pain disorder (DMS-III(R)) can rarely be made accurately, or else with the new criteria attaching to it will reflect uncertainty of explanation rather than a conversion condition.

group of patients in whom pain had no detectable physical cause and who were known to have psychiatric illness. Sternbach and Timmermans (1975) have also reported that when pain was effectively treated personality changes occurred for the better. Irritability or aggression have a biological purpose in connection with pain. If pain is due to assault by an aggressor, it is helpful to have some type of subjective or overt response to combat the attack. Irritability is one such response. Its frequent occurrence in the context of chronic pain is thus quite understandable.

Merskey et al. (1987) have shown that a relationship exists between individuals' perception of their childhood experience and chronic pain. They also found that patients with chronic pain did not have any particular relationship with hysteroid or obsessoid traits. However, obsessoid or introverted individuals had a significant but weak tendency to score more highly on scales for anxiety, depression and irritability.

These findings imply that depression, anxiety and irritability will be most prevalent in patients who have either a painful lesion or premorbid introverted/obsessoid characteristics. Since the latter relationship is definite but not strong and much depression and anxiety were found in pain clinic patients who had organic lesions it is plausible to suppose that the major relationships between pain and depression, in a variety of pain clinics which the authors studied, are the consequence of pain causing depression rather than vice versa.

Finally, in this section it is worth noting that schizophrenia is often associated with a reduction in subjective complaints of pain and that of all psychiatric illnesses it seems to have the lowest rate of complaints of pain, both those of physical origin and those of psychological origin (Watson et al, 1981). Some of the instances of pain due to psychological causes in schizophrenia may, however, be of particular interest and deserve further exploration. They have been relatively little studied to date.

References

Ahles, T. A., Yunus, M. B. and Masi, A. T. (1987) Is chronic pain a variant of depressive disease? The care of primary fibromyalgia syndrome. *Pain*, **29**, 105–111

American Psychiatric Association (1987) *Diagnostic and Statistical Manual*, 3rd edn (Revised). APA, Washington, D.C.

Banks, M. H., Beresford, S. H. A., Morrell, D. C. et al. (1975) Factors influencing demand for primary medical care in women aged 20–40 years; a preliminary report. *International Journal of Epidemiology*, **4**, 189–255

Crook, J. and Tunks, E. (1985) Defining the 'chronic pain syndrome': an epidemiological method. In: *Advances in Pain Research and Therapy* (eds

H. L. Fields, R. Dubner and F. Cervero), Raven Press, New York, pp. 871–877

Fishbain, D. A., Goldberg, M., Meagher, R. et al. (1986) Male and female chronic pain patients categorized by DSM-III psychiatric diagnostic criteria. *Pain*, **26**, 181–189

Gould, R., Miller, B. L., Goldberg, M. A. et al. (1986) The validity of hysterical signs and symptoms. *Journal of Nervous and Mental Disorders*, **174**, 593–587

International Association for the Study of Pain (Sub-committee on Taxonomy) (1979) Pain terms: a list with definitions and notes on usage. *Pain*, **6**, 249–252

Melzack, R., Wall, P. D. and Ty, T. C. (1982) Acute pain in an emergency clinic: latency of onset and descriptor patterns related to different injuries. *Pain*, **14**, 33–43

Merskey, H. (1965) The characteristics of persistent pain in psychological illness. *Journal of Psychosomatic Research*, **9**, 291–298

Merskey, H., Lau, C. L., Russell, E. S. et al. (1987) Screening for psychiatric morbidity. The pattern of psychological illness and premorbid characteristics in four chronic pain populations. *Pain*, **30**, 141–158

Mitchell, S. Weir (1872) *Injuries of Nerves and Their Consequences*. Dover, New York

Naliboff, B. D., Cohen, M. J. and Yellen, A. N. (1982) Does the MMPI differentiate chronic illness from chronic pain? *Pain*, **13**, 333–341

Romano, J. M. and Turner, J. A. (1985) Chronic pain and depression: does the evidence support a relationship? *Psychology Bulletin*, **97**, 18–34

Spear, F. G. (1967) Pain in psychiatric patients. *Journal of Psychosomatic Research*, **11**, 187–193

Sternbach, R. A. (1974) *Pain Patients. Traits and Treatment*. Academic Press, New York

Sternbach, R. A. and Timmermans, G. (1975) Personality changes associated with reduction of pain. *Pain*, **1**, 177–181

Tyrer, S. P., Capon, M., Peterson, D. M. et al. (1989) The detection of psychiatric illness and psychological handicaps in a British pain clinic population. *Pain*, **36**, 63–74

Watson, G. D., Chandarana, P. C. and Merskey, H. (1981). Relationships between pain and schizophrenia. *British Journal of Psychiatry*, **138**, 33–36

Watson, D. (1982) Neurotic tendencies among chronic pain patients: an MPPI item analysis. *Pain*, **14**, 365–385

Weeks, R., Baskin, S., Rapoport, A. et al. (1983) A comparison of MMPI personality data and frontal electromyographic readings in migraine and combination headache patients. *Headache*, **23**, 75–82

Woodforde, J. M. and Merskey, H. (1972) Personality traits of patients with chronic pain. *Journal of Psychosomatic Research*, **16**, 167–172

5

Psychiatric and psychological issues in different illnesses

S. P. Tyrer

Certain illnesses and certain locations for pain have been found to be associated with a greater than expected frequency of emotional problems. Walters (1961) purported that pain arising from the head and neck was more likely to have little evidence of organic pathology to account for it compared with pain arising from other parts of the body, particularly the limbs. These findings have been reported consistently. The aim of this chapter is to discuss the psychiatric and psychological factors that are found in particular illnesses where chronic pain is a feature.

Headache

Headache can arise from a large number of different causes. These include nervous and muscle tension, changes in the blood supply, e.g. migraine, anything that causes increased intracranial pressure, e.g. cerebral tumour, subarachnoid haemorrhage and trauma to the head, even when this is relatively mild. Many chronic headaches are precipitated and maintained by emotional factors but it is important to accurately exclude any treatable cause before assuming that a headache is entirely accounted for by psychological or psychiatric factors.

Chronic tension headache

Two types of tension headache have been described. The first type consists of a sensation of a continuous band round the head or pressure which tends to last throughout the day on most days and is not affected to any extent by analgesics. The second type tends to be more intermittent, often occurs on one side of the face, lasts a few hours only and the affected areas are tender to touch. Analgesics are usually helpful for a few hours.

The first type of headache is strongly influenced by emotional factors and is associated with a feeling of being on edge or nervously keyed-up or strained. It may be due to alteration in cerebral blood flow or of changes in nerve conduction although the exact mechanism is not established. The second type of headache is due to excessive contraction of muscles of the scalp and head and is similar to the muscle pains that occur after extreme exercise.

Both headaches are common when there is emotional tension and when the experience of headache is relatively short lived (less than 18 months) antidepressants may be of help. These should not be administered as a blanket prescription but only after determining what factors are associated with the headaches. This is much easier to determine with the second type of headache because of its intermittent nature. Advice on how to deal with sources of tension and how to avoid these may be sufficient to ameliorate the problem. It is important to exclude treatable causes such as refractive errors of vision leading to eye strain.

Migraine

Migraine headache is over-diagnosed. There are two forms of migraine, classical and common migraine. In classical migraine there is uni-lateral, throbbing head pain usually preceded by a visual stimulus like scintillating lights. Pain usually lasts from four to ten hours if drugs are not taken but may last up to 24 hours. In common migraine there is no aura prior to the headache occurring and the headache usually last from one to three days but may last longer. It may not be unilateral.

The earlier investigators of migraine headache found that many of their patients were ambitious and rigid and found it difficult to express resentment. More recent studies have shown that these patients are not typical of the majority of patients with migraine but are more representative of patients who go to a specialized clinic for treatment of their problem. Patients who have a combination of migraine and muscle contraction are more likely to be preoccupied with their pain and have some degree of depression. Some patients with common migraine have muscle contraction headaches and, if these are pro-longed, they are more likely to have distress. This seems to be related to persistence of pain.

Cluster headache

Cluster headache, sometimes known as migrainious neuralgia, consists of unilateral pain mainly occurring on the front and sides of the head occurring in separate bouts with often daily attacks for several months. It is usually associated with watering of the eyes and/or nose. It is not associated with particular personality or psychiatric factors although patients with chronic symptoms can become demoralized.

Post-traumatic headache

Between 30 and 50% of all people who injure their heads sufficiently to need admission to hospital develop chronic post-traumatic headaches. In most of these patients there are no gross neurological defects but disturbance of convergence of vision, poor coordination and balance, nystagmus, dilatation of the retinal vessels and temporary EEG changes are found in many patients. There are frequent psychiatric symptoms that occur at the same time. These mainly involve irritability, inability to concentrate, light headedness and poor tolerance of alcohol.

The general consensus is that these 'psychiatric' symptoms are due to the minimal brain damage that is sustained during the injury. In the majority of cases there is no evidence of a psychiatric syndrome presenting and subjects have been found to have normal MMPI profiles. In some cases, particularly when the incident that caused the trauma was of an unexpected nature, patients develop symptoms of anxiety associated with memories of the event causing the injury, which can be sufficiently intense to justify the diagnosis of post-traumatic stress disorder. This is said to be present if the patient re-experiences the trauma by intensive recollections or dreaming, is unable to re-establish his former interests and shows numbing of his response to others. Associated symptoms include exaggerated startle response, guilt and sleep disturbance. There is some evidence that patients who develop this disorder have predisposing vulnerable personalities. There is sometimes a good response to amitriptyline.

Orofacial pain

Pain in the region of the mouth and face may be due to a large number of causes. Pain may arise from the teeth and related structures, the mucous lining of the mouth and throat, salivary glands, blood vessels, nerves and joints. There are two forms of facial pain where no recognizable physical cause can be found to account for pain, atypical odontalgia, where there is persistent throbbing pain in the teeth, and oral dysaesthesia or burning tongue syndrome.

Atypical odontalgia

Atypical odontalgia was until recently largely described under the label of atypical facial pain. In this condition pain is felt deep in the soft tissues of the bone and is usually throbbing in nature with the teeth being hypersensitive to stimuli. Patients may be excessively concerned with oral hygiene. At least four out of five patients with this condition presenting for treatment are females. No consistent organic findings have been found in this condition. It is possible that the pain in this condition is due to excessive grinding of the teeth (bruxism) or that there is a primary vascular disturbance in the periodontal region.

Patients with atypical odontalgia complain of frequent psychiatric symptoms and their MMPI profiles are psychopathological. They are difficult to treat but there is sometimes considerable benefit obtained by giving antidepressants to these patients. Lascelles (1966) showed that the monoamine oxidase inhibitor, phenelzine, had a gratifyingly beneficial effect in three-quarters of patients with this condition. Others have not found quite such good results but recent trials have shown that tricyclic antidepressants that increase the availability of serotonin are effective in this condition (Feinmann, Harris and Cawley, 1984). It has been suggested that this syndrome is a form of depression masquerading in the form of chronic pain. This may be so, although it is difficult to test.

Oral dysaesthesia

Oral dysaesthesia or burning tongue syndrome, like atypical odontalgia, is four times commoner in women than in men. The tip and lateral borders of the tongue are normally involved and there is often a disturbance of taste, dry mouth and intolerance of dentures. It is customary for there to be relief of pain by eating and drinking. These patients have a normal oral mucosa on examination. The burning sensation continues throughout the day.

Unlike atypical odontalgia a physical cause can often be found in this condition. Aetiological factors include deficiency of iron, folic acid or vitamin B_{12}, raised fasting blood glucose concentrations, and thrush, a fungal infection of the mouth. Associated symptoms are increased thrusting of the tongue and subjective reduced salivary gland flow.

In some of these patients tricyclic antidepressants are effective. It is important to consider all factors that could contribute to this syndrome before embarking on psychological or psychiatric treatments.

Temporomandibular pain and dysfunction syndrome

Temporomandibular pain dysfunction syndrome, sometimes known as myofascial pain dysfunction syndrome, includes the following features:

1 Pain and tenderness on palpation of the muscles involved in chewing, the masticatory muscles.

2 Limitation of movement of the mandible, and

3 Sounds from the temporomandibular joint during movements of the lower jaw.

A surprisingly large percentage of the population (10–15%) suffer from this syndrome with or without arthritis of the temporomandibular joint. Again, as for atypical facial pain, the incidence of the syndrome is much more frequent in female patients, although this may be because they seek help more than males.

Early work emphasized the contribution of psychological factors to this illness. Many authors underlined the increase in anxiety, depression and conversion hysteria in this group of patients. However, as with migraine, more recent enquiry has shown that patients with temporomandibular pain show little neuroticism compared with control subjects and there is little evidence of personality abnormality. There is a group of patients with this disorder who are more likely to be psychologically disturbed. These are patients whose symptoms have arisen following injury to the jaw. This is probably related to the fact that the prognosis of this condition when there is jaw injury is not as good as when it arises from some other non-traumatic cause. If there is no jaw injury the outcome of patients treated compared with those untreated is not significantly different, symptoms improving considerably within a three-month period. However, tricyclic antidepressants often help, and re-education and exercise of the masticatory and neck muscles may also be of benefit. Correction of occlusal bite was recommended by earlier authors but there does not appear to be a strong rationale for this treatment.

The change in presentation of this illness, similar to that of migraine, suggests that this common disorder is associated with significant personality abnormalities and psychiatric symptoms in only a minority of patients. Years ago, hypochondriacal patients were the main attenders at clinics concerned with this illness, which was first described in 1934 by Costen, and it is the contact with these patients that may have persuaded the earlier investigators to think that the origin of this illness was largely psychological or psychiatric. Present evidence suggests there is a group of patients with this disorder, some of whom have developed this after jaw injury, who are over-preoccupied and concerned about their pain. However, in the majority of cases there is no evidence of major psychological distress and the disorder is self-limiting.

Disorders of the neck

Cervical sprain syndrome

This illness results from forcible hyperextension of the neck, often following a collision in which a motor vehicle is struck from the rear. The victim complains of a dull aching pain in the back of the head or neck and a trigger point, focal tenderness over a palpable taut band of muscle fibres, can usually be felt outside the painful area. Although in the majority of cases the patient experiences relief from pain within three months, in a group of patients the symptoms may persist or even increase. Although a number of these patients are involved in compensation claims, and this may contribute to disability, settlement of the issue does not usually produce corresponding improvement in the patient's physical state (*see* Chapter 6). These patients may become very demoralized because of their inability to work, there is often marital friction and accompanying depression resulting from the chronic painful state can occur. The reason why these patients become more ill than their brethren is probably related to more severe joint and soft-tissue injury, muscle spasm, vertebral artery involvement or damage to the labyrinth. This syndrome is one of a group of myofascial pain disorders and is discussed more fully later in this chapter.

Chronic abdominal pain

Peptic ulcer

Peptic ulcers occur in both the stomach and the duodenum. Duodenal ulcers occur twice as frequently as gastric ulcers. The occurrence of duodenal ulcers is to some degree related to stress factors although a clear relationship has not been consistently shown. It has been suggested that patients who develop duodenal ulcers are more likely to be driving, perfectionist personalities and have difficulty in adapting to change. Again, as with migraine and temporomandibular joint disease the more representative the population of patients with duodenal ulcers studied, the more they show normal personality characteristics. It is likely that a large number of factors are involved in the precipitation of duodenal ulcers of which stress is an important one, with possibly some contribution from personality structure.

Irritable bowel syndrome

This syndrome consists of chronic abdominal pain in many parts of the abdomen but with the greatest frequency over the left lower quadrant of the abdomen. The pain is associated with an alteration in bowel habit, usually in the form of diarrhoea, although constipation occurs. In many of these patients there is a history of previous abdominal pain and dysmenorrhoea in women.

Although there is undoubtedly increased motility of the lower gastrointestinal tract, which may be associated with increased sensitivity to gastrointestinal hormones such as cholecystokinin and to prostaglandins, psychiatric factors are more prominent in this illness than in most abdominal diseases. Patients with irritable bowel syndrome have higher anxiety and are more introverted than patients with other abdominal complaints or patients with ulcerative colitis, a disease that has a large psychosomatic component. Some have described them as pain-prone. Although no studies have shown that the increase in anxiety is a consequence of the bowel problem or is a cause of it many patients have had evidence of high anxiety before developing disordered bowel function. It is known that raised tension causes an increase in the rhythmic contractions of muscle in the large bowel, so the fact that high anxiety is associated with this illness may be as a result of the anxiety rather than the cause. Relaxation is beneficial.

Ulcerative colitis

Ulcerative colitis is a more serious disease than irritable bowel syndrome. The symptoms are similar to irritable bowel syndrome in that bouts of lower abdominal pain occur associated with nausea and loose stools. However, unlike irritable bowel syndrome, the stools contain blood and mucus. It has been found that high arousal, e.g. anxiety, anger or ecstasy can precipitate bouts of loose stools in these patients.

In general, it is found that patients who develop abdominal pain and have few organic findings have a family history of similar type, e.g. dyspepsia. In addition, it is found that in a substantial number of patients that the onset of their abdominal pain has occurred following some major life event. This is often the death of a close member of the family (*see* Chapter 3).

Pelvic pain

The main causes of chronic pelvic pain are menstrual abnormalities, endometriosis, damage or structural abnormalities of the supporting structures of the uterus, chronic pelvic inflammatory disease, pain from urinary tract structures, colonic or rectal pain and ovarian pain. Pain due to menstrual abnormalities tends to be episodic. Dysmenorrhoea refers to pain that occurs during menstruation itself and in the majority of women over the age of 30 who present with this condition the cause is due to endometriosis, a condition where ectopic areas of endometrial tissue are found outside the uterus, and fibroids. Pain in premenstrual tension occurs a week before periods are due and is not normally the major complaint. It is common for pelvic pain to increase in the premenstruum in many conditions and cyclical pain of this sort should not automatically be assumed to be due to endometriosis or hormonal abnormalities.

In the main, the organs in the pelvis are not acutely sensitive to pain. Pain occurs where there is displacement of structures, e.g. retroversion of the uterus, pelvic inflammatory disease or carcinoma.

In some women with chronic pelvic pain there is no clear organic cause. This syndrome has recently been re-classified by the International Association for the Study of Pain as chronic pelvic pain without obvious pathology (CPPWOP). Lower abdominal pain with, less frequently, low back pain are the presenting symptoms and on examination tenderness is elicited in the reproductive structures, particularly the uterus and supporting ligaments. Deep dyspareunia, or pain on intercourse, is common.

Although most patients with CPPWOP are in psychological distress the studies that have been performed do not show any clear differences in personality between patients with this syndrome compared with other women with chronic pain of known aetiology. Although there is a group of these patients where there is a history of dependent personality characteristics and previous sexual abuse, the majority of women who present with this condition do not exhibit characteristic psychological or psychiatric features. Pelvic circulatory disturbance or damage to the supporting structures of the uterus resulting from surgical operation or damage following pregnancy, may explain some of the symptoms in these patients. Pelvic pain is not at all clearly localized or understood and CPPWOP should not be regarded as a condition in which psychological or psychiatric factors predominate. This condition should not be diagnosed definitely without a negative laparoscopy.

References

Feinmann, C., Harris, M. and Cawley, R. (1984) Psychogenic facial pain: presentation and treatment. *British Medical Journal*, **288**, 436–438

Lascelles, R. G. (1966) Atypical facial pain and depression. *British Journal of Psychiatry*, **112**, 651–659

Walters, A. (1961) Psychogenic regional pain alias hysterical pain. *Brain*, **84**, 1–18

Bibliography

Bass, C. (ed.) (1990) *Somatisation—Physical Symptoms and Psychological Illness.* Blackwell Scientific Publications, Oxford.

6

Chronic pain and compensation

G. Mendelson

The complaint of chronic pain is frequent among both the recipients of workers' compensation payments, and personal injury litigants. The clinician involved in the management of such patients is often required to testify as to the relationships between the complaint of persistent pain, the extent of impairment, the continuing payment of benefits, and the likely effect of termination of such payments and finalization of litigation on the patient.

Pain is a subjective experience, and thus particularly difficult to assess in the adversarial situation which often develops in the context of litigation and compensation. Because additional damages may be awarded for 'pain and suffering' in common law litigation, it is not infrequently claimed that plaintiffs—as well as recipients of compensation payments—complain of pain when it is not present or tend to exaggerate its severity so as to maximize their damages or benefits. There is no empirical evidence for such an allegation (Mendelson, 1987a).

It is necessary to utilize a systematic approach to the assessment of a litigant with a chronic pain complaint. The clinician should evaluate any possible predisposing and personality factors that may contribute to the development of chronic pain and, if possible, arrive at a diagnosis of the cause of the pain complaint (*see* Chapter 7).

This chapter will review studies exploring the relationships between the accident compensation system and both the presentation and the duration of chronic pain complaints. The effect of compensation and litigation on the treatment response of chronic pain patients, as well as comparisons of the pain experience and description of chronic pain patients involved in litigation or receiving compensation and those without such involvement will also be examined.

The compensation system and chronic pain

In examining the influence of compensation on chronic pain, it is helpful to compare populations which have different systems of compensation and litigation. It is fortuitous that New Zealand, in 1974, adopted a universal system of compensation for injuries. Under this system

1 the traditional workers' compensation scheme was abolished;

2 the right to sue in civil courts at common law for personal injuries was abolished;

3 a new scheme was established to provide benefits to all who suffer an injury, irrespective of fault or circumstances; and

4 the new scheme was universal in that it covered all persons in New Zealand (Sandford, 1979).

Two published studies have examined the characteristics of chronic pain patients in New Zealand with those in countries which continue to have the traditional workers' compensation systems and maintain the right to sue at common law for personal injuries. Carron, DeGood and Tait (1985) compared patients attending pain clinics in the United States with those in New Zealand. Mills and Horne (1986) compared patients with the so-called 'whiplash' injury (cervical sprain syndrome) in New Zealand with those in Victoria, Australia.

Carron, DeGood and Tait (1985) compared the pain and disability ratings of patients referred for treatment, and attempted to relate the treatment outcome to the type of compensation or disability benefits received by the patients in the two countries. The Accident Compensation Commission in New Zealand meets the full cost of medical care, and provides income security, for all accident victims irrespective of fault, thus avoiding litigation with its concomitant 'adversary' system within which many personal injury cases are played out.

The authors found that, at the time of the initial visit to the pain clinic, 49% of the US sample and 17% of the NZ sample were receiving pain-related compensation. A significantly greater proportion of US patients reported sleep disturbance, reduced social and recreational activities, and impaired libido. On follow-up, although the US compensation patients reported a greater level of subjective improvement, they reported the highest degree of pain intensity and frequency, the greatest limitation of activities, and the lowest return to full activity and ability to work. It was noted that 'the differential effects linked to compensation status are quite small, and almost non-existent in the NZ sample.'

Carron, DeGood and Tait concluded that the difference between

Table 6.1 Characteristics of 'whiplash' injuries in New Zealand and Victoria*

	New Zealand	Victoria
Rear-end collisions	547	2,181
Number of 'whiplash' injuries	422	4,231
'Whiplash'/rear-end collision	0.77	1.94
Mean compensation	NZ $1038	Aust. $3265

*From Mills and Horne (1986).

the patient groups in the two countries was related to the no-fault system in New Zealand, which automatically provided income compensation for accidental injury without the need to prove injury at work, and the consequent absence of an adversarial relationship between the claimant, employer and insurer.

Mills and Horne (1986) obtained statistics for the 12-month period to 30 June 1983, and analysed the number of motor vehicle accidents, rear-end collisions, claims for 'whiplash' injuries, and the mean compensation paid to each claimant. The results of the comparison is shown in Table 6.1.

In commenting on these findings, the authors noted that 'the striking difference in the incidence of whiplash injury in the two groups suggests that litigation and the expectation of financial compensation may have an influence on development of whiplash symptoms.'

Mills and Horne suggested further that 'because patients in Victoria would seek compensation for an injury through the common law system ... they are more conversant with and more attuned to receiving compensation for injury, which may in itself be stimulus for claiming for an injury that they would not normally have claimed for,' whereas that stimulus 'does not exist in New Zealand.'

These authors also analysed the statistics for 'time off work' of the two patient groups. Data was available for 227 cases in New Zealand, and for 1558 cases in Victoria. Of the New Zealand group, 212 (93.4%) returned to work within six months; the comparable figure for Victoria was 1126 (72.3%). This difference is statistically significant.

The relationship between societal expectations concerning illness and illness behaviour was explored by Balla (1982) in an analysis of the 'late whiplash syndrome' as manifested in Australia and Singapore. The 'late whiplash syndrome' was defined as a condition which follows a motor vehicle accident, usually after a rear-end collision. The injured person complains of persistent pain and other symptoms, long after the acute pain resulting from the soft-tissue injury would have been expected to subside. The typical syndrome includes neck pain and stiffness, headache, pain in the arms, problems in carrying out usual daily activities, sleep disturbance, and loss of libido. Other symptoms include irritability, anxiousness, poor memory and concentration, and feelings of depression.

Analysis of the socio-demographic characteristics of 300 patients, examined in Australia, with the 'late whiplash syndrome', with pain and other symptoms persisting for longer than six months after the accident, showed that there were very significant associations between this condition and 'social structural markers'. It was found that it occurred more often in the upper-middle occupational brackets, and the age distribution was in the 30–50 year groups in males and 20–40 year groups in females, whereas motor car accident statistics indicated that these predominantly involve younger age groups, particularly among males. It was also noted that migrants of Northern and Central European background were over-represented among the patients.

Balla attempted to compare the characteristics of patients with the 'late whiplash syndrome' from Singapore, with those seen in Australia. He reported that this condition 'was unheard of' in Singapore 'but for the odd case seen in those with European backgrounds'. A prospective study of 20 patients with an acute whiplash injury, whose 'original acute complaints of pain in the head and neck region were the same as seen in Australia', found that the symptoms resolved and did not go on to develop the 'late whiplash syndrome'.

Balla concluded, on the basis of his findings, that the 'late whiplash syndrome' is a 'culturally constructed illness behavior based on indigenous categories and social structural determinants'. He also noted that in Australia such a condition has been accepted as compensable by the courts, and that this provides a positive reinforcement for 'illness behavior' following the acute phase of 'whiplash'. He also noted that as there are 'no clear and frequent precedents' in Singapore following a whiplash injury, this was 'likely to be one explanation for significant differences in behavior in association with an illness which may have taken place'.

The effect of compensation on response to treatment

Most authors report that continuing compensation payments have an adverse effect on the recovery rate. It has been noted that one aspect of compensation payments is to perpetuate symptoms and disability because of an adverse effect on the recipients' self-esteem and the promotion of dependency.

Studies of the effect of compensation on treatment outcome of chronic pain, published prior to 1983, were in general agreement that patients in receipt of compensation and/or involved in litigation had a worse prognosis than those with similar complaints who were not in receipt of such payments nor involved in litigation (Mendelson, 1983).

Aitken and Bradford (1947) reported on 170 patients operated on for a ruptured disc following an industrial injury. They did not have a comparison group, but in reporting the overall poor result of surgical treatment commented that 'the desire for financial reimbursement for injuries received...has definitely influenced the end result'.

Other studies have compared treatment responses of similar groups of patients receiving pain-related compensation payments with those not compensated. Krusen and Ford (1958) reported on 509 patients with low back injuries, and noted that 56% of 272 patients receiving disability payments improved with treatment, as compared with 89% improvement among the 237 patients not receiving compensation.

Another representative study was that by Gurdjian et al. (1961), who reported a follow-up of 915 patients operated on for herniated lumbar intervertebral discs. They found that among those in receipt of pain-related compensation 'excellent and good results' were obtained by between 61.5 and 50% (depending on the surgical procedure), as compared with 76.6 and 72.5% respectively among those not in receipt of compensation.

However, Reynolds, McGinnis and Morgan (1959), in a study of 115 patients operated on for low back pain and sciatica found that there was no difference in outcome between those receiving compensation and those with no medicolegal involvement.

The presence or absence of litigation was also one of several factors considered by Gore and Sepic (1984) when evaluating the results of cervical disc fusion in a group of 146 patients. There was no significant correlation between presence or absence of litigation and improvement following surgery.

Catchlove and Cohen (1983) have compared the return to work rates of a group of 20 pain patients claiming compensation—who were treated without any specific instruction concerning resumption of work—with that of a group of 27 patients who received similar treatment at a pain clinic but who also had been given a specific 'return to work as part of the therapy' instruction.

The two groups were compared on variables such as age, sex, pain duration, site of pain, and treatment duration, and no significant difference between the two groups was found. However, among the 'instruction' group 16 out of the 27 patients (59%) returned to work during treatment at the Pain Management Unit, whereas among the 'no instruction' group 5 out of 20 patients had resumed work (25%). Follow-up data was obtained for 15 patients in each of the two groups. Of 10 patients in the 'instruction' group who had returned to work and were available for follow-up a mean of 9.6 months after termination of treatment, 9 were continuing to work; among patients from the 'no instruction' group 3 out of 4 were working a mean of 19.9 months after treatment ceased.

The authors of this study commented that at times the direction to return to work was met with 'rage and anger and even, on occasion, personal threats against the therapist'. However, patients who did return to work showed a sense of satisfaction and increased independence. It was concluded that a directive approach of this type was an important part of the 'holistic' treatment of patients with chronic pain receiving workers' compensation.

Dworkin et al (1985) have reported a study involving 454 chronic pain patients, in which the influence of employment and compensation on treatment outcome was examined by a multiple regression analysis. The results showed that those who were working at the time of entry into the treatment programme had a better response to treatment than non-working patients, and that patients receiving compensation had a poorer short-term treatment response than those not receiving compensation, but only employment was a statistically significant predictor of long-term outcome.

The authors of this study concluded that it was important to direct attention 'toward the roles of activity and employment in the treatment and rehabilitation of chronic pain patients', within the individual's limitations. They also commented on the 'deleterious effects' of terms such as 'compensation neurosis' which are used to label patients and which may direct attention away from the need to involve the patient in an active treatment programme.

Sander and Meyers (1986) compared the period of work disability following a low back sprain/strain injury among two groups of patients, drawn from railway employees covered by a Federal disability scheme in the United States. One group consisted of those injured while at work, and the other comprised those injured off duty. The two groups were matched for type of injury, and for gender.

The authors found that those injured on duty (and hence receiving compensation benefits) were away from work for a mean of 14.2 months, as compared with 4.9 months for those injured off duty. This difference was statistically significant, and the authors concluded that 'the financial rewards of compensation' were responsible for the prolonged recovery of those injured at work. This study demonstrated a worse short-term prognosis for return to work among workers in receipt of pain-related compensation.

Comparison studies

An early study which compared the pain behaviour of litigants with that of non-litigants was undertaken by Peck, Fordyce and Black (1978). Although deserving mention as this was the first published comparison of pain characteristics between two patient groups, this study is open to criticism on the grounds that both patient groups were in receipt of compensation, the difference between them being the presence of an additional tort claim.

A different method of comparison between patients with chronic low back pain receiving compensation and those who had no such claims was described by Leavitt et al (1982). These authors compared the two groups on pain measures such as duration, intensity, locus of pain, pain description, and the quality of pain. The groups consisted of 85 patients receiving compensation, and 176 patients not on compensation and with no pending claims.

The results of the comparison indicated that patients who had objective evidence of injury but showed no significant psychological disturbance, and were receiving compensation, reported more intense sensory discomfort. However, no other differences between the compensation and non-compensation groups was found. The difference in the sensory discomfort rating may have been due to an over-emphasis of the actual initial injury.

Pain ratings, using the McGill Questionnaire and the visual analogue scale, were recorded by 80 patients with chronic low back pain, who had been referred for assessment and/or treatment at a pain clinic (Mendelson, 1984b). The patients were divided into two groups according to whether or not they were claiming compensation, and the groups compared with respect to psychological and pain variables. At the time of the initial evaluation 47 patients were in receipt of compensation payments and involved in litigation, whereas 33 patients were not receiving compensation, had not been involved in pain-related litigation, and were not entitled to any form of compensation.

Patients in the 'compensation' group tended to be younger (mean 37.1 years, range 18–58 years) than the patients in the 'non-compensation' group (mean 41 years, range 25–61 years). Patients in the 'compensation' group had a significantly shorter mean duration of pain (33.6 months, range 8–144 months) than in the 'no compensation' group (mean 114.2 months, range 6–420 months).

In a comparison the various measures of pain severity, the visual analogue scale scores, and the mean scores on the categories of the McGill Pain Questionnaire checklist failed to demonstrate any significant difference in either the severity or the characteristics of low back pain described by the 'compensation' group and the 'no compensation' group. Within each of these two groups there was no correlation between pain duration and pain severity.

The role of compensation in chronic pain was also examined by Melzack, Katz and Jeans (1985). These authors reported on a group of 145 patients with chronic pain of at least six months' duration, who had been referred to the Pain Clinic at the Montreal General Hospital. There were 81 patients with chronic low back pain (of these, 27 were receiving compensation and 54 were not). Sixty-four patients had musculoskeletal pain, mainly affecting the upper back, shoulders, or lower limbs (of these 15 were on compensation and 49 were not). In describing the patients who were in receipt of compensation payments, the authors do not specify whether or not the patients were also involved in litigation.

The patients in this study were an unselected consecutive sample of Pain Clinic referrals. Analysis of results for the low back pain group showed that there was a 'remarkable consistency with which low-back pain patients describe their pain—regardless of whether or not they receive financial compensation for their illness'.

Analysis of results for the musculoskeletal pain group showed that compensation patients subjectively evaluated the overall pain intensity as lower than the non-compensation group; the compensation group had also sought the opinion of fewer consultants. Thus, contrary to the common notion of pain exaggeration by litigants, in this group of patients those involved in litigation described the pain as less severe, when compared with a group not involved in litigation.

Discussion

Studies reviewed in this chapter indicate that: (1) the prevalence of chronic pain complaints is positively correlated with compensation systems which provide pain-contingent benefits and allow litigation at common law; (2) compensation and litigation often have an adverse effect on treatment response in chronic pain, but this effect is modified by work and by the provision of specific treatment programmes; and (3) there is no evidence to support the view that chronic pain patients involved in litigation or receiving compensation describe their pain as more severe or more distressing than similar patients with pain which is not compensable.

Although not directly pertinent to this chapter, it is perhaps worth noting that patients with chronic pain receiving compensation or involved in litigation do not, as has been asserted by some authors, invariably improve and return to work following the finalization of the claim. Research refuting this assertion has been summarized elsewhere (Mendelson, 1984a; Sprehe, 1984).

In reviewing the literature dealing with chronic pain and compensation, one of the problems encountered is that of lack of specificity in the description of the compensation, litigation, and work status of the patient groups. The study by Dworkin et al. appears to be the only one to have distinguished between those recipients of compensation payments who were working, and those who were not. The finding that work status in this group of chronic pain patients was an important predictive factor of treatment outcome makes it important for future studies to consider employment status as a separate variable.

The studies by Balla (1982), Carron, DeGood and Tait (1985), and Mills and Horne (1986) emphasize that the assessment of chronic pain patients needs to take into consideration societal expectations, and that attitudes to illness and illness behaviour must also be considered. However, using the Illness Behaviour Questionnaire no difference between litigants and non-litigants with chronic pain was demonstrated (Mendelson, 1987b).

The impact of the compensation system and of litigation on the process of becoming a chronic pain patient has important social policy implications which until now has been neglected by governments and by policy-makers.

The studies comparing the pain description by litigants with that of non-litigants do not support the frequent assertion that patients claiming compensation describe their pain experience as more severe than a comparable group of pain patients not seeking compensation payments. The only study to find a significant difference between the two groups was that of Leavitt et al. (1982), who showed that litigants with objective evidence of injury, and no evidence of significant psychological disturbance, reported more intense sensory discomfort. The authors suggested this may have been the result of an over-emphasis on the symptoms of the actual initial injury among patients who may have considered that the injury was 'not regarded with sufficient seriousness by the employer'.

There is also no evidence to support the view that litigants with chronic low back pain are significantly more psychologically disturbed than similar patients not claiming compensation (Mendelson, 1984b). This finding contradicts the view that patients involved in litigation develop the specific psychological condition termed 'accident neurosis' or 'compensation neurosis', as these patients could not be distinguished on psychometric testing from those not seeking compensation. Dworkin et al. have specifically commented on the deleterious effect of using such labels, which have no clinical validity (Mendelson, 1985).

As shown by Fishbain et al. (1988), both male and female patients with chronic pain receiving compensation are more likely to be diagnosed as having a Conversion Disorder (somatosensory type) than similar patients not receiving compensation. Male patients in receipt of compensation were more likely to be given a diagnosis of one of the Personality Disorders than similar patients not receiving compensation. The authors suggested that the finding with respect to Conversion Disorder may be due to the intervening variable of socio-economic status. The finding with respect to prevalence of personality disorder may reflect the tendency of those with premorbid difficulties in meeting the demands of work and social functioning to experience particular difficulty in returning to their preinjury level of functioning.

However, the study by Fishbain et al. did not find any evidence of a specific clinical picture such as 'compensation neurosis', and the diagnosis of Generalized Anxiety Disorder was significantly more frequent among female chronic pain patients in the 'non-compensation' group.

The findings reviewed in this chapter suggest that the effect of compensation on chronic pain complaints can best be conceptualized as occurring at an unconscious rather than a conscious level, as do other secondary gains which tend to perpetuate psychogenic symptoms (Merskey, 1979). This emphasizes the need to carefully evaluate each litigant with chronic pain to assess the relative importance of compensation and other factors, and to avoid stereotyping or labelling litigants as generally motivated by potential financial gain.

Consideration of the social policy implications of the relationship between compensation, litigation and chronic pain is outside the scope of this review. However, it is relevant to note that the studies cited above indicate that where litigation and/or continued compensation payments are dependent on ongoing work disability, the complaint of chronic pain often becomes the 'badge' of such continuing work incapacity and, as such, resistant to treatment. Most compensation systems are adversarial in nature, and the resulting combination of anger, resentment, bureaucracy, entitlement attitudes, and peer group expectations create a climate in which the complaint of chronic pain persists long after the initial physical cause has resolved.

It has been shown that specific treatment programmes can reduce the likelihood of progress to chronicity following work injuries. Fordyce et al. (1986) and others have shown that a treatment programme for low back pain, which incorporates behavioural methods, is more effective than traditional management. Thus, the effect of compensation on treatment response can be modified by specific programmes which stress early mobilization and return to the work-place, appropriate activity and exercises, and avoidance of other factors which may promote 'learned pain behaviour' (Tyrer, 1986). Factors which influence outcome following compensable injury have been summarized in Table 6.2.

The New Zealand experience is still too scanty to allow any but tentative conclusions about the effect of a no-fault accident compensation system on the rate of chronic pain and work incapacity. However, if the findings of Carron, DeGood and Tait (1985), and of Mills and Horne (1986) are confirmed by future studies, then it will seem clear that such policy reforms have an important role in the prevention of chronic pain and work incapacity following industrial and motor car injuries.

Table 6.2 Factors influencing outcome following injury

Developmental: physical/sexual abuse
              emotional deprivation
              childhood hospitalization

Personality: hypochondriacal traits
           dependency
           obsessionality
           passive-aggressive

Cultural: folk beliefs concerning disease
        illness behaviour

Work factors: job dissatisfaction
            occupational stress

Psychological reaction to injury: altered self-concept
                              altered body image
                              personality disorganization
                              regression

Interpersonal changes: within family
                  within social milieu

References

Aitken, A. P. and Bradford, C. H. (1947) End results of ruptured intervertebral discs in industry. *American Journal of Surgery*, **73**, 365–380

Balla, J. I. (1982) The late whiplash syndrome: a study of an illness in Australia and Singapore. *Culture, Medicine and Psychiatry*, **6**, 191–210

Carron, H., DeGood, D. E. and Tait, R. (1985) A comparison of low back pain patients in the United States and New Zealand: psychosocial and economic factors affecting severity of disability. *Pain*, **21**, 77–89

Catchlove, R. and Cohen, K. (1983) Directive approach with Workmen's Compensation patients. *Advances in Pain Research and Therapy*, **5**, 913–918

Dworkin, R. H., Handlin, D. S., Richlin, D. M. et al. (1985) Unraveling the effects of compensation, litigation, and employment on treatment response in chronic pain. *Pain*, **23**, 49–59

Fishbain, D. A., Goldberg, M., Labbe, E. et al. (1988) Compensation and non-compensation chronic pain patients compared for DSM-III operational diagnoses. *Pain*, **32**, 197–206

Fordyce, W. E., Brockway, J. A., Bergman, J. A. et al. (1986). Acute back pain: a control group comparison of behavioral vs. traditional management methods. *Journal of Behavioral Medicine*, **9**, 127–140

Gore, D. R. and Sepic, S. B. (1984) Anterior cervical fusion for degenerated or protruded discs: a review of one hundred forty-six patients. *Spine*, **9**, 667–671

Gurdjian, E. E., Webster, J. E., Ostrowski, A. Z. et al. (1961) Herniated lumbar intervertebral discs — an analysis of 1176 operated cases. *Journal of Trauma*, **1**, 158–176

Krusen, E. M. and Ford, D. E. (1958) Compensation factor in low back injuries. *Journal of the American Medical Association*, **166**, 1128–1133

Leavitt, F., Garron, D. C., McNeill, T. W. et al. (1982) Organic status, psychological disturbance, and pain report characteristics in low-back-pain patients on compensation. *Spine*, **7**, 398–402

Melzack, R., Katz, J. and Jeans, M. E. (1985) The role of compensation in chronic pain: analysis using a new method of scoring the McGill Pain Questionnaire. *Pain*, **23**, 101–112

Mendelson, G. (1983) The effect of compensation and litigation on disability following compensable injuries. *American Journal of Forensic Psychiatry*, **4**, 97–112

Mendelson, G. (1984a) Follow-up studies of personal injury litigants. *International Journal of Law and Psychiatry*, **7**, 179–188

Mendelson, G. (1984b) Compensation, pain complaints, and psychological disturbance. *Pain*, **20**, 169–177

Mendelson, G. (1985) 'Compensation neurosis': an invalid diagnosis. *Medical Journal of Australia*, **142**, 561–564

Mendelson, G. (1987a) Measurement of conscious symptom exaggeration by questionnaire: a clinical study. *Journal of Psychosomatic Research*, **31**, 703–711

Mendelson, G. (1987b) Illness behaviour, pain and personal injury litigation. *Psychiatric Medicine*, **5**, 39–48

Merskey, H. (1979) *The Analysis of Hysteria*. Baillière Tindall, London

Mills, H. and Horne, G. (1986) Whiplash – manmade disease? *New Zealand Medical Journal*, **99**, 373–374

Peck, C. J., Fordyce, W. E. and Black, R. G. (1978) The effect of the pendency of claims for compensation upon behavior indicative of pain. *Washington Law Review*, **53**, 251–278

Reynolds, F. C., McGinnis, A. E. and Morgan, H. C. (1959) Surgery in the treatment of low-back pain and sciatica: a follow-up study. *Journal of Bone and Joint Surgery*, **41A**, 223–235

Sander R. A. and Meyers, J. E. (1986) The relationship of disability to compensation status in railroad workers. *Spine*, **11**, 141–143

Sandford, K. L. (1979) Five years of accident compensation. *New Zealand Medical Journal*, **90**, 257–258

Sprehe, D. J. (1984) Workers' compensation: a psychiatric follow-up study. *International Journal of Law and Psychiatry*, **7**, 165–178

Tyrer, S. P. (1986) Learned pain behaviour. *British Medical Journal*, **292**, 1–2

Part Two

Assessment and Intervention

7

Assessment measures

S. P. Tyrer

The assessment of the patient with chronic pain includes the evaluation of physical, psychological, social and cultural factors. It is vital to assess the contribution of all these dimensions in the assessment of chronic pain. A comprehensive assessment, therefore, involves obtaining a clear description of the nature of the pain, previous personality and level of medical and psychological functioning as well as an accurate evaluation of current disabilities. The emphasis of this chapter is concerned with the psychiatric and psychological assessment of patients with chronic pain. However, an assessment of this nature cannot be carried out in isolation; the nature of any past and current physical problems should be addressed first and the emotional component of the complaint of pain evaluated after the extent of physical pathology has been ascertained. There are advantages if the physician assessing the psychological and psychiatric contribution to the pain complaint is also experienced in the assessment of physical factors leading to chronic pain. This is the exception rather than the rule but in a multidisciplinary pain clinic, with different practitioners able to consult each other on site, the patient should be confident that all aspects of his painful complaint are being considered by the appropriate experts.

Throughout, the clinician should be constantly aware of the dimensions involved in the manifestation of pain as described in Chapter 3. These include nociception, the stimulation of sense organs in the periphery that are concerned with identifying noxious stimuli, perception of pain in the brain, evaluation of its meaning and pain behaviour. It is the latter two dimensions with which the psychologists and psychiatrists will be primarily concerned although the meaning of their assessment will be dependent on the contribution of pain from the first two dimensions.

Factors in history and examination

At first assessment, as full a record as possible of all past treatments and interventions should be obtained. The results of any investigations that have been carried out on the patient should be at hand and these should be explained to the patient in language that he can understand. A good deal of anxiety is caused by erroneous evaluation of symptoms by patients. Information given to them by doctors or nurses in hospitals is also often misinterpreted and may be the source of considerable anxiety.

It is helpful to ask the patient what he believes is the cause of both his present and past pains. Many patients describe their pains using medical terms which have different meanings to the patient and doctor. For example, the word 'arthritis' has been described to me by separate patients as 'a grinding down of all the bones' and as 'stiffening of the joints so that they lock together and you cannot get them unstuck'.

An accurate account should be obtained of the circumstances surrounding the onset of the pain. How far did it follow physical damage, either from injury or from disease? Even when there is a clear organic cause for the pain, it is important not to overlook the psychological and psychiatric state of the patient at the time injury or disease occurred or was recognized. There are a number of major incidents that occur in people's lives that are associated with emotional illness. These include all occurrences involving a major loss to the person, including death of a person close to the patient, loss of a job or divorce. However, other major changes that are normally considered as positive factors, including getting married or bearing a child may sometimes have adverse emotional consequences because of the change in adjustment required.

Enquiries should be made about the intensity of the pain. If the patient is familiar with the Visual Analogue Scale or Pain Line, illustrated in Figure 1.3, p. 14, they should be asked the level of their pain at the time of interview on a scale of 0–10. It is also valuable to ask how much the pain fluctuates during the day and whether the intensity of the pain has increased since the pain complaint started, remained the same or been variable. When patients are in distress from physical or psychiatric factors they tend to rate the intensity of their pain as higher. Patients who say their pain is gradually increasing over time sometimes have pronounced psychological distress as a result of the demoralizing effects of chronic pain but physical factors may also contribute.

Questions that should be addressed about the nature of the patient's pain are illustrated in Table 7.1. Pain that is accurately localized in particular dermatomes, that is described with such adjectives as sore, boring or nagging, that is exacerbated markedly by particular

Table 7.1. Questions to ask about the patient's pain

When did your pain first start?

Where do you feel your pain?

When does your pain occur?

How intense is your pain?

How does it change throughout the day?

What is the effect of movement and change in posture on your pain?

What other factors (a) make your pain worse?
(b) make it better?

What do you now do less frequently and what do you do more frequently since you developed the pain?

Does your mood affect your pain?

What effect do drugs have on your pain?

movements and which is sufficient to wake the patient from sleep is likely to be associated with an organic cause. However, the converse is not necessarily true. It is now known that pain that is imprecisely described and affects circumscribed regions of the body may have physical origins. Pains that affect whole regions of the body, e.g. the whole leg or a single arm were thought to have a psychogenic cause but recent work by Gould and his colleagues (1986) has shown that these pains often have an organic aetiology.

This being said, pain that occurs in multiple sites in the body, that has increased in area over time, which is described as frightful, dreadful or punishing, which is not affected by specific movements, that does not wake the patient from sleep and which is barely affected by analgesic drugs or by physical treatments such as transcutaneous electrical nerve stimulation (TENS), is more likely to be found in patients who have a substantial contribution from psychological and psychiatric factors to their pain.

After the history, the patient should be examined. If the psychiatrist carries out this procedure it will help to give him a much better understanding of the extent of organic factors that are contributing to the painful complaint. Patients are also more likely to accept explanations about the origin of their pain from a doctor who has examined them. Warning signs that have been associated with non-organic pathology include over-reaction to examination, weakness of all muscle groups in a particular region of the body, superficial tenderness, production of pain when manoeuvres are employed which the patient thinks will cause pain but in fact do not affect body mechanics, e.g. pressure on head, and variable performance when distracting tests are used, e.g. increased ability to straight leg raise when examining a patient whilst sitting (Waddell et al., 1980).

However, the examiner must beware of attributing a psychogenic cause to the patient's pain on the basis of inappropriate signs on examination. It is unfortunately frequent for physicians to erroneously diagnose hysteria in patients who exhibit physical signs that do not appear to obey anatomical precepts. Gould and colleagues (1986) have shown that apparent hysterical signs on examination are found frequently in patients with organic illness and their presence does not indicate that pain arises from psychogenic sources. However, if there is a considerable disparity between symptoms and signs this should encourage the examiner to look for factors other than physical ones to explain them.

At this stage, the doctor should have a reasonable idea of the physical diagnosis and how pain and other symptoms are affecting the patient's life. It is useful to ask a number of questions about the pain at this point. These include:

1 Is there evidence of existing physical disease or past tissue damage?

2 If so, has pain persisted beyond the time that healing would have been expected to take place?

3 Is there evidence of psychiatric illness, and if this is present is it primary or secondary?

4 Are there any emotional conflicts or psychosocial problems that were associated with the onset of the pain or with its continued maintenance?

5 Is there any suggestion of intentional production or feigning of symptoms?

A good deal of knowledge of the patient's past history, previous personality, recent life events and conflicts, and other social and cultural factors are needed to determine how far these are affecting the production of the painful complaint. For these reasons, the most difficult question to answer immediately is the fourth. A suggested schema to help in the assessment of pain problems is illustrated in Figure 7.1.

This figure is only a guide. The inexperienced observer is inclined to over-emphasize the contribution of organic pathology in individuals who complain of persistent pain. However, as psychiatrists are used to examining for evidence of psychiatric illness and many patients with chronic pain are in psychological distress, there is a tendency once the examiner has seen a number of patients with chronic pain to underrate the extent of organic factors in causing pain. Virtually all patients have contributions from organic, psychiatric, personality and sociocultural factors in determining their response to chronic pain and the skill of the pain therapist is in evaluating the extent of

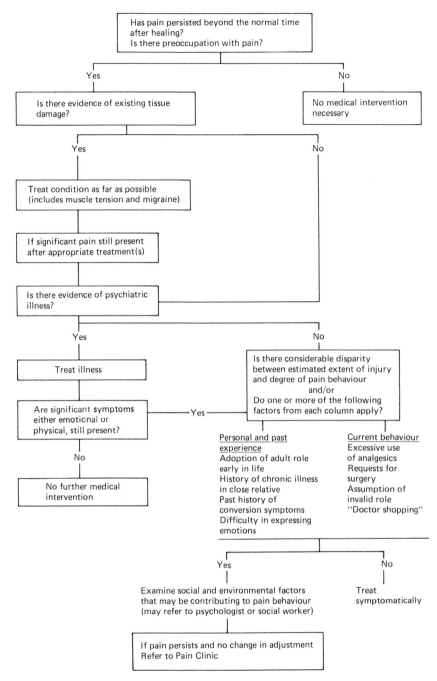

Figure 7.1 *Schema for assessment of psychological and psychiatric factors in chronic pain.*

these components. To aid him in this task, the following techniques, investigations and instruments can be used.

Assessment instruments

Description and intensity of pain

Three main major classes of words have been found to describe pain, sensory, emotional and intensity. Adjectives to describe pain that fall into the sensory category include burning, crushing, sharp, sore and throbbing. Words that have an emotional or affective quality comprise agonizing, dreadful, exhausting, punishing and sickening. The intensity of pain is described by words such as weak, moderate, strong, intense, severe and excruciating. A check-list of 78 words describing pain states, the McGill Pain Questionnaire, is widely used in this context (Melzack, 1975).

The number of words selected on the McGill Pain Questionnaire is most closely associated with the intensity of the pain felt. It is not too surprising that it is in these cases that psychological distress is most apparent. Although patients who use a greater number of affective or mood-related pain words are more likely to rate positively on psychological and psychiatric scales for distress and illness, this relationship is not very close.

Cognitive Factors

The significance attached to the sensation of pain depends upon its meaning to the sufferer. Constant pain following an operation is interpreted differently from similar pains that arise de novo. The patient's own appraisal of the extent to which pain interferes with previously desired activities and subsequent feelings of helplessness and reduced self-control has been found to predict the development of depression and disability. These findings are important; they tell us that it is not the severity of disease or intensity which determines the degree of disability but the beliefs of the patient about how far this is the case. In particular, the beliefs that pain is going to endure, that its cause is unknown and uncertainty about its effect lead to demoralization and depression.

The doctor's attitude and reaction to the patient's assumptions is crucial. In addition to providing a satisfactory explanation for the pain and the prognosis of the condition the physician should try and understand and acknowledge the extent of the pain and the limitation this causes. The patient's perceptions may be faulty because he has pain but the physician is often biased in the opposite direction because he is pain-free and may never have experienced extreme pain. Physicians recovering from operations have found that the doctors looking after them had much less serious an opinion about the severity of their patient's pain than the sufferer. The physician can do no worse than remember an old Arab saying about a man experiencing severe toothache who describes his pain as being worse than two thousand dead in Jerusalem.

During the history and examination of the patient inaccurate beliefs about the origin and duration of the pain should have been identified. However, if a more precise evaluation of faulty thoughts and beliefs about pain is required this can be obtained by administering the Cognitive Errors Questionnaire (Smith et al. 1986). This is helpful if specific attention is proposed to alter cognitions in a structured way (see Chapter 11).

Psychiatric factors

There are three main ways in which psychiatric illness can be manifest in the form of pain, in hysterical or hypochondriacal ways, in the context of a depressive illness and occasionally as part of a delusory system.

Many patients with chronic pain are found to exhibit elements of hysterical and hypochondriacal mechanisms. Hysterical in this context means the exhibition of a symptom or loss or reduction in physical functioning which suggests physical disorder but cannot be explained entirely on a physical basis. It is rare, however, for patients to have the full syndromes of conversion hysteria or of hypochondriacal neurosis. It is rather that with a symptom such as pain, which cannot be observed by another, attempts to explain the symptom to others results in behaviour which may be interpreted as hysterical or hypochondriacal. At the time of the first symptoms, the patient will usually have been examined in detail and investigations carried out. He usually has been led to believe that he has a physical illness and the investigations will show what this is. If pain persists in the absence of abnormal laboratory and radiological investigations further tests are likely to be made which further reinforce the patient's opinion that there must be something wrong. If after all these procedures no diagnosis can be made the patient is understandably frustrated and further symptom exaggeration and non-organic signs may develop. Understandably the full triad of symptoms in hypochondriacal neurosis—persistent belief of illness, fear of the illness, and preoccupation with bodily symptoms—is not usually found. Most patients are convinced that they have an organic disease but it is rare for them to be fearful of this and indeed the opposite is usually the case. Patients are almost always relieved if they are told that they have a particular disease, as long as this is not progressive and does not affect mortality in the short-term. Even if there is no treatment for the disease condition they are pleased with this information. 'I always knew there was something wrong, doctor. Now you have put my mind at rest'.

When hysterical and hypochondriacal symptoms and signs are present they will be detected during the history and examination. The assessment of behaviour resulting from these mechanisms is considered in the subsequent section on pain behaviour.

Depression is frequently associated with chronic pain. Between 30% and 40% of patients attending chronic pain clinics can be categorized as suffering from depressive illness according to well-established schedules for the diagnosis of depression. It is helpful both for the physician and the patient to determine how far a depressive illness is due to the secondary effects of pain or whether it is a primary phenomenon. If there is weight loss, guilt and social withdrawal primary depression is more likely to be the diagnosis and antidepressants may be more likely to help these individuals. The dexamethasone suppression test (DST), which involves the administration of dexamethasone the previous night followed by measurement of serum cortisol levels taken on one or two occasions the following day, has been found to distinguish patients with major depression from those without (France and Krishnan, 1985). This test would be valuable if those with increased serum cortisol (non-suppressors) were found to be responsive to physical treatments for depression. Although there is a suggestion this is so this issue has not been examined in detail in patients with chronic pain. Positive DST results occur in a wide variety of illnesses including anorexia and dementia and the initial enthusiasm for this test has waned.

Self-rating and observer depression instruments can help in the diagnosis of depression in this population. The most efficient and customary way of using these questionnaires is to employ the self-rating scales as screening instruments to detect emotional factors and to interview in depth those who score highly on these. The Beck Depression Inventory (Beck et al. 1961) and the General Health Questionnaire (GHQ) (Goldberg, 1972) have been widely used in this area.

If cognitive treatment is available the Beck scale is valuable as cognitive symptoms in depression are well represented amongst the items in this instrument. Patients scoring fifteen or more, particularly if those questions concerned with cognitive factors are emphasized, may benefit from a referral to a psychologist or psychiatrist. The GHQ has some utility but a higher cut-off point (above 11 on the 28-item questionnaire) needs to be used in identifying patients with chronic pain who have psychiatric disturbance than in a general population sample. This is not surprising; a number of the symptoms directly associated with chronic pain are also prime symptoms in depressive illness. For instance, many patients with chronic pain complain of poor sleep, feel slowed up and are irritable because of their pain.

To avoid the contamination of these physical factors in the assessment of depression Zigmond and Snaith (1983) developed the Hospital Anxiety and Depression (HAD) Scale. Because of its design, this questionnaire may have greater utility than many in assessing depression in this population. The forerunner of this scale, the Leeds Scale for Anxiety and Depression, was found to provide the best discrimination between psychiatric and non-psychiatric cases amongst four widely used self-assessment schedules (Tyrer et al., 1989). However, in common with other scales designed for assessment of patients with chronic illness a higher cut-off score for the identification of depression and anxiety needs to be used if the HAD is used as a screening instrument. Preliminary analysis in the Newcastle Pain Relief Clinic shows that the diagnostic confidence of this instrument is best when the cut-off score is 11/12 for depression and 13/14 for anxiety. The sensitivity of this scale using these criteria was 86%, in a sample of 100 patients.

Observer rating scales for depression in chronic pain by contrast are rarely used except for research purposes. It may be simpler to ask for specific symptoms of illness. Identification of depression in general practice has been reliably predicted if at least one positive response is made to questions concerned with low energy, loss of interests, loss of confidence and feelings of hopelessness (Goldberg et al., 1988). Another schema that may be employed to help in diagnosis is the administration of the operational criteria of the Diagnostic and Statistical Manual for Mental Disorders, Third Edition (Revised) (DSM-III R) (American Psychiatric Association, 1987), ideally by using the Structured Clinical Interview for DSM-III (R) (SCID) (Spitzer et al., 1988).

Occasionally, an acutely psychotic patient may complain of pain because of his beliefs. The classic case of the man who believed he was Jesus Christ on the road to Calvary and complained of pain in a band around his forehead is an example. The mechanism of pain in such cases is easily elicited as long as an adequate history can be obtained.

Muscle tension can of course give rise to pain and many patients attending Pain Clinics have pain from this source. Many are found to have bands of contracted muscles and the term 'myofascial pain syndrome' has been used to describe patients with this complaint. Although there is some relationship between psychic anxiety and myofascial disease, this relationship is not close. Assessment by physical examination is of more value in these cases than using instruments to assess anxiety.

Pain behaviour

Although what patients say about the severity of their pain and the degree to which they have reduced their previous activities are related, direct observation does not usually closely reveal a close association between these measures. The best way of determining behaviour is for observers to directly record the amount of time a person lies down, sits, stands and partakes in various activities. It is not usually feasible to carry this out successfully in normal clinical practice and it has been shown that if the subject himself records this behaviour at hourly intervals on an appropriate form then a reasonably good approximation can be made of actual activities.

Opinions vary about whether pain levels should be recorded on such forms. One disadvantage of this is that the patient is encouraged to concentrate on their pain throughout the day. However, it is a valuable assessment exercise at the start of treatment to determine what factors are associated with amelioration of pain and which activities make it worse. This exercise also enables the clinician to directly challenge faulty statements by the patient, e.g. 'in the afternoons, my pain couldn't be worse', when their recorded diary shows that there are many occasions when the listed pain is not of maximum intensity. An example of a pain diary is illustrated in the Appendix, page 201.

Other information that can be usefully obtained include the frequency of visits to doctors, admissions to hospital and the number of operations. These all represent manifestations of pain behaviour, whether this is justified or not. High figures in any of these categories is associated with increased disability and distress and a poorer prognosis.

Pain behaviour at interview can be measured by counting the number of times the subject grimaces, limps and guards his body (Keefe and Hill, 1985). Although this is a reliable and valid measure of pain behaviour such recordings only indicate the extent of this measure when the patient is in contact with the health care specialist. This may not be representative of their degree of pain behaviour elsewhere. In their own home, the patients' pain behaviour may be encouraged by their spouse or family, and previous experience and personality factors may also lead to exhibition of this behaviour. Assessment of this aspect of the behaviour is not easy but information from a close family member can often provide useful pointers towards this.

Questionnaires are of limited value in this area. The Illness Behaviour Questionnaire (IBQ) (Pilowsky and Spence, 1975) has been widely used, and is able to distinguish clearly the self-reported beliefs and behaviour of patients attending a chronic pain clinic from those seen in general practice settings. However, the instrument is unable to distinguish patients with chronic pain and psychiatric difficulties from those who have fewer emotional problems. A shorter version of this questionnaire has been recently designed and needs to be evaluated. A much simpler assessment instrument of function that indirectly measures pain behaviour is the Self Care Assessment Schedule (Benjamin et al., 1984).

A number of instruments have been developed which assess behavioural, cognitive and mood measures at the same time. A widely used example is the West Haven–Yale Multidimensional Pain Inventory (WHYMPI) (Kerns, Turk and Rudy, 1985). The reliability and validity of these instruments are still undergoing assessment but they may usurp many of the scales evaluating more discrete items.

Predisposing factors to psychiatric illness in chronic pain

Certain social, economic, cultural, past history and personality features predispose towards individuals developing a chronic painful state. These were suggested as early as 1895 by Breuer and Freud. In 1959 Engel described a group of patients whom he regarded as 'pain-prone'. These patients were termed masochistic in that they seemed to court disaster, they had a history of numerous unsuccessful operations and they were chronically guilt-ridden. In the background of these individuals there was often a history of parental abuse, either physical or emotional, in which the expression of pain by the child was one of the few ways to gain a response from the parent. A typical example was a parent who punished his or her child frequently but then suffered remorse and overcompensated with affection so that the child became accustomed to the sequence of pain and suffering being followed by love. The importance of these observations was that physicians dealing with chronic pain began to enquire about emotional factors as well as physical ones when they saw their patients. Engel's views were all the more influential as he was both a Professor of Medicine as well as a Professor of Psychiatry.

Most patients attending pain clinics do not fall within Engel's 'pain-prone' group. There are patients who have been brought up in families where chronic illness of at least one family member has been the norm and where minor illnesses and disability are followed by weeks away from work and/or expressions of illness. It is not surprising that a child brought up in such a household often models such behaviour he has observed when he experiences similar problems as an adult. There is another group of patients who are highly work-orientated and who are disproportionally distressed when pain prevents them carrying out their former activities. Manual workers and those with dissatisfying jobs tend to report more pain than white-collar workers.

The assessment of these factors is important to the physician both in terms of treatment and prognosis. When a full history is obtained it is clearer why patients have reacted in the way they have to adversity and illness.

The personality characteristics of patients developing chronic pain have been widely studied. However, most of the investigations have described personality features in patients who have been in pain for some years. Chronic pain affects attitudes and beliefs and the personality characteristics assessed at the time of long-standing pain may not represent the previous personality type of the sufferer. It is unfortunate that most of the studies of personality in patients with chronic pain have been made using the Minnesota Multiphasic Personality Inventory (MMPI). The MMPI scales were designed originally to apply to patients with psychiatric illness and no physical illness. Pain and disability are associated with elevated scores on the Hypochondriasis, Hysteria and Depression subscales of this instrument. Previously it had been thought that this inverted V pattern on the graphed profile of the MMPI represented a personality type that was prone to develop chronic pain but in fact this is a result of having a chronic disability.

The problem of disentangling the effects of chronic pain on the personality of the patient from the patient's pre-morbid state makes it difficult to make solid pronouncements on the personality type of patients who are prone to develop chronic pain. Studies have suggested that individuals with dependent and passive-aggressive personalities are found more frequently in pain clinics and there are theoretical grounds for assuming that introspective personalities may also be pain-prone. Some patients have a hypochondriacal personality disorder. Characteristics of this include excessive preoccupation with maintenance of health, magnification of minor ailments, repeated medical consultation and rigid beliefs about health.

Patients that somatize their mental distress, i.e. who present with physical symptoms when there is emotional conflict, can present to pain clinics. A subgroup of these patients may have major difficulties in expressing their feelings; the term 'alexithymia' has been used to describe these individuals (Sifneos, 1973).

Some patients who value their physical prowess are prone to become very distressed when they sustain an injury or develop an illness which prevents them from exercising their bodies in their customary way. These individuals have been described as suffering from 'Athlete's Neurosis' (Little, 1969). A number of patients seen in pain clinics fulfil the criteria for this description, which is often associated with a poor prognosis.

Future studies need to determine the personality of the patient before illness developed. This can be measured by using the Personality Assessment Schedule which relies on information provided by a close informant (Tyrer and Alexander, 1988).

Factors affecting response to treatment

A number of factors that render individuals vulnerable to chronic pain also adversely affect their response to treatment. Those who are unemployed at the beginning of treatment, who are receiving compensation before treatment is given and who do not receive treatment until many years after the onset of their pain, have a poor prognosis in terms of their pain disability. Somatizers, i.e. people who express their emotional distress as physical symptoms also do poorly. At the other end of the spectrum, patients who complain of a multitude of psychiatric symptoms also do not do well. Religious faith and good educational attainment are associated with better adjustment.

Ultimately, successful adaptation to chronic pain depends upon the sufferer accepting the extent and handicaps due to his pain and recognizing that his own efforts are of greater importance than those of the doctors and other pain clinic professionals in improving the quality of his life. The degree to which this measure can be assessed is one of the functions of instruments that measure locus of control for beliefs. A number of these exist and that by Wallston, Wallston and DeVellis (1978) can be recommended.

Conclusion

The assessment instruments chosen to evaluate the emotional factors in chronic pain depend above all on the clientele that attend the clinic and the facilities that are available. An adequate history and examination is by far the most important part of assessment but valuable additional information can be obtained by means of questionnaires and schedules.

The instruments described are not necessarily helpful in determining specific treatment. This can best be decided after all information is available. They are useful as a baseline measure of symptoms and functioning and can also help in determining prognosis and the intensity of intervention by professional staff. Symptoms and beliefs should be assessed separately.

The most useful questionnaires are the HAD scale as a screening test to detect depression and anxiety (Zigmond and Snaith, 1983), and the WHYMPI (Kerns, Turk and Rudy, 1985) for the behavioural assessment of pain. An assessment of activity is useful and can either be assessed directly or by means of a pain diary. Locus of control questionnaires (Wallston, Wallston and DeVellis, 1978) are helpful in both determining outcome before applying behavioural techniques and to determine ultimate prognosis.

References

Beck, A. T., Ward, C. H., Mendelson, M. et al. (1961) An inventory for measuring depression. *Archives of General Psychiatry*, **4**, 561–571

Benjamin, S., Barnes, D., Falconer, G. et al. (1984) The effect of illness behaviour on the apparent relationship between physical and mental disorders. *Journal of Psychosomatic Research*, **28**, 387–395

Engel, G. (1959) 'Psychogenic' pain and the pain-prone patient. *American Journal of Medicine*, **26**, 899–918

France, R. D. and Krishnan, K. R. R. (1985) The dexamethasone suppression test as a biological marker of depression in chronic pain. *Pain*, **21**, 49–55

Goldberg, D. P. (1972) The detection of psychiatric illness by questionnaire. *Maudsley monograph No.* 21, Oxford University Press, London

Goldberg, D. P., Bridges, K., Duncan-Jones, P. et al. (1988). Detecting anxiety and depression in general medical settings. *British Medical Journal*, **297**, 879

Gould, R., Miller, B. L., Goldberg, M. A. et al. (1986) The validity of hysterical signs and symptoms. *Journal of Nervous and Mental Disease*, **149**, 593–597

Keefe, F. J. and Hill, R. W. (1985) An objective approach to quantifying pain behaviour and gait patterns in low back pain patients. *Pain*, **21**, 153–161

Kerns, R. D., Turk, D. C. and Rudy, T. F. (1985) The West Haven-Yale Multidimensional Pain Inventory (WHYMPI). *Pain*, **23**, 345–356

Little, J. C. (1969) The athlete's neurosis—a deprivation crisis. *Acta Psychiatrica Scandinavica*, **45**, 187–197

Melzack, R. (1975) The McGill Pain Questionnaire; major properties and scoring methods. *Pain*, **1**, 277–299

Pilowsky, I. and Spence, N. D. (1975). Patterns of illness behaviour in patients with intractable pain. *Journal of Psychosomatic Research*, **19**, 279–287

Sifneos, P. (1973) The prevalence of 'Alexithymic' characteristics in psychosomatic patients. *Psychotherapy and Psychosomatics*, **22**, 255–262

Smith, T. W., Aberger, E. W., Follick, M. J. et al. (1986) Cognitive distortion and psychological distress in low back pain. *Journal of Consulting Clinical Psychology*, **54**, 573–575

Spitzer, R. L., Williams, J. B. W., Gibbon, M. et al. (1988). Instruction manual for the Structured Clinical Interview for DSM-III-R. New York: Biometrics Research

Tyrer, P. and Alexander, J. (1988) Personality Assessment Schedule. In *Personality Disorders: Diagnosis Management and Course* (ed. P. Tyrer), Wright, Bristol, pp. 43–62

Tyrer, S. P., Capon, M., Peterson, D. M. et al. (1989) The detection of psychiatric illness and psychological handicaps in a British pain clinic population. *Pain*, **36**, 63–74

Waddell, G., McCulloch, J., Kummel, E. et al. (1980) Non-organic physical signs in low back pain. *Spine*, **5**, 117–125

Wallston, K. A., Wallston, B. S. and DeVellis, R. (1978) Development of the Multi-dimensional Health Locus of Control (MHLC) scales. *Health Education Monographs*, **6**, 160–170

Zigmond, A. S. and Snaith, R. P. (1983) The hospital anxiety and depression scale. *Acta Psychiatrica Scandinavica*, **67**, 361–371

8

Psychotropic drugs

J. W. Thompson and S. P. Tyrer

Psychotropic drugs are those which affect mental function; the word comes from two Greek words *psuke* = soul or mind and *tropos* = a turn. They are used very widely and in the UK in 1985 there were 31 203 000 prescriptions of psychotropic drugs. Those psychotropic drugs used are indicated in Table 8.1.

History of use of psychotropic drugs for chronic pain

The field of psychopharmacology is a very new one. Until 1952 the only drugs that affected mental processes were sedatives like barbiturates and paraldehyde, some antihistamines and preparations containing bromides. These drugs had no useful specific action on the

Table 8.1. **Classification of Psychotropic Drugs**

Group	Example
Antidepressants	amitriptyline (tricyclic)
	trazodone (non-tricyclic)
	phenelzine (MAOI)
Antipsychotics	chlorpromazine
synonyms	haloperidol
major tranquillizers,	
neuroleptics	
Minor tranquillizers	
synonyms	
anxiolytics, sedatives	
Hypnotics	temazepam
Anti-manic drugs	lithium carbonate
synonyms	carbamazepine
mood normalizers	
Psychostimulants	dexamphetamine
Psychodysleptics	lysergic acid diethylamide (LSD)
	cannabis

brain other than sedation. In 1952 the modern psychopharmacological era started with the discovery of chlorpromazine, which, although sedative in large doses, specifically ameliorates the symptoms of schizophrenia. The development of antidepressants followed within the next few years and the benzodiazepine group of drugs for anxiety and lithium for the control of mood states also started to be widely used at this time.

The earliest reference to the use of psychotropic drugs for treatment of chronic pain was in 1956 by Margolis and Jianascol. Although chlorpromazine has some analgesic action in acute pain, a greater effect was shown after administration of imipramine which was the first antidepressant synthesized. Imipramine is actually closely related chemically to chlorpromazine. These two classes of drugs have remained the mainstay of psychotropic treatment for chronic pain.

Reference should also be made to the drug carbamazepine and other drugs with similar properties such as phenytoin and sodium valproate. These drugs are normally classified as anticonvulsants because they are effective in the treatment of epilepsy. Their use antedates the development of chlorpromazine. Recently it has been found that these drugs are useful in a variety of mood states and in reducing aggression and hyperactivity. Although they are not usually considered under the heading of psychotropic drugs, the effectiveness of these agents has been demonstrated in a number of psychiatric conditions like mania and overactivity and it is therefore very appropriate to consider them under the psychotropic heading.

The evidence for the efficacy of each group within this class of drugs in chronic pain will be considered separately for each group.

Antidepressants

Antidepressant drugs such as amitriptyline and imipramine have been used for the treatment of chronic pain since shortly after their ability to improve mood in depressed subjects was first found in 1958. It is known that these drugs increase the amount of certain monoamines in the central nervous system, allowing an increase in neurotransmission along mood-related pathways in the brain. There is evidence that in some types of depression, there is a diminution of monoamines, in particular serotonin or 5-hydroxytryptamine. Serotonin plays an important role in the control of pain pathways in the brain (see Chapter 1). Thus pain behaviour can be reduced by electrical stimulation of neurones in the central part of the brain which contains substantial amounts of serotonin. Conversely, removal of these areas from the brains of animals makes them particularly sensitive to painful stimuli. Furthermore, the close relationship between serotonin and the endorphins and enkephalins in nerves involved in the transmission of painful stimuli makes it likely that agents which reduce available serotonin are also likely to reduce endorphin release with consequent increase in the effect of substance P (*see* Chapter 1). The converse also holds true; increased activity in nerves where endorphins or enkephalins are the neurotransmitters will result in an increase in available serotonin.

Numerous studies have now been carried out which show that antidepressants have a clear benefit in reducing pain in patients with chronic pain syndromes. Although the relief of pain sometimes results because the antidepressant improves an associated depression, there are a number of factors which indicate that in many cases these drugs do not exert their action simply by relieving depression. Thus patients who suffer from chronic pain but who are not depressed may also benefit from antidepressant drugs. In other patients who are clearly depressed, antidepressants reduce the level of pain without any amelioration of the depression. Of even greater significance is the fact that antidepressant drugs used in doses lower than those known to be effective in the treatment of depression, produce an analgesic effect.

The antidepressant drugs that have been studied most widely in chronic pain are the tricyclic antidepressants. Since these are also the mainstay of conventional antidepressant treatment, they have also been the most widely studied in this context. Because of the relationship between serotonin and pain relief, it is reasonable to expect that those drugs which have a substantial effect on serotonin should also be the most effective in chronic pain. For this reason, drugs that have this effect have come under special scrutiny. Amitriptyline and dothiepin, which both exert their action by facilitating nerve transmission along serotonin pathways, have both been found effective in reducing pain independently of their antidepressant action. Watson et al. (1982) in Canada showed that amitriptyline was effective in patients with post-herpetic neuralgia who were free of depression when compared with inactive drug treatment. Feinmann, Harris and Cawley (1984) in London found dothiepin to be an effective treatment in patients with facial pain. It appears therefore that antidepressant drugs which substantially influence serotonin have an analgesic action. However, other drugs that have substantially less effect on serotonin, such as desimipramine and imipramine, have also been found to be helpful in chronic pain. It has also been suggested that antidepressants with an intact tertiary amine structure, e.g. amitriptyline and clomipramine, sometimes called the methylated antidepressants, are more effective in promoting analgesia than the demethylated drugs like nortriptyline. It is said that the methylated antidepressants have more pronounced effects on serotonin but there is no clinical evidence that this is the case. Antidepressants have many other effects in addition to their action on amines and their ability to alter the distribution of receptors (up regulation) involved in neurotransmission may be much more important in explaining their effects.

The monoamine oxidase inhibitors (MAOIs), the other main group of antidepressants that were discovered at about the same time as the tricyclic antidepressants, have been less widely used in the treatment of pain states. This reflects their relative lack of use compared with the tricyclic antidepressants, which is partly consequent upon the adverse effects they cause when certain foods are taken with these drugs. However, there are good theoretical grounds for supposing that they will be effective in pain as they cause an increase in release of all monoamines. The most comprehensive study of their use was by Lascelles in London in 1965 (Lascelles, 1966). He showed that 30 out of 40 patients improved during administration of phenelzine. Most of these patients were depressed to some degree and the improvement in their pain was associated with a concurrent alleviation in their depression. Many patients with facial pain do not complain of depression although careful enquiry can reveal symptoms that occur in depressive illness. In these cases exhibition of phenelzine can sometimes have a dramatic effect.

Newer drugs that specifically inhibit serotonin re-uptake and consequently increase the amount of available amine are now being developed for the treatment of depression. The results of experimental work suggest that these should be of value in the treatment of chronic pain and the results of clinical trials are awaited with eagerness. These drugs include fluvoxamine, fluoxetine and trazodone.

Antipsychotics

The antipsychotic agents or major tranquillizers are widely used in the treatment of both acute and chronic pain although the evidence for their efficacy is limited. In acute pain nearly all phenothiazines have an *anti*-analgesic effect half an hour after first administered although later they do have some effect in diminishing pain sensation. However, the only drug that has an established place in the treatment of chronic pain is methotrimeprazine. This has been shown to decrease cancer pain in well-controlled studies and, when given with drugs like morphine, can reduce the dose of opiate required. Unfortunately methotrimeprazine, more so than most phenothiazines, can cause profound hypotension. A different neuroleptic called flupenthixol, a member of the thioxanthene group, decreases the duration, intensity and frequency of chronic tension headaches when given orally in low doses. This effect may be secondary to an anxiolytic action.

The antipsychotic drugs block dopamine receptors in the limbic system, an area of the brain concerned primarily with emotional responses. Although these drugs cause some decrease in anxiety, this is not their primary mode of action and any analgesic effect they possess is probably not mediated by these means. It seems likely that they alter the patient's emotional response to pain by some other mechanism.

Anticonvulsants

In 1885 the famous French neurologist Trousseau noted that the paroxysms of pain in trigeminal neuralgia bore a striking resemblance to epilepsy and he called it 'epileptiform neuralgia'. More than 50 years later this led Bergougignan to carry out a successful trial of phenytoin in 1942. In 1962 Blom introduced carbamazepine for the treatment of trigeminal neuralgia, again with success. It is therefore hardly surprising that both of these drugs have been used in the treatment of chronic pain arising in other parts of the body. To a large extent, phenytoin has been superseded by newer drugs such as carbamazepine, sodium valproate and clonazepam.

This group of drugs inhibit the firing of central or peripheral nerve impulse generators and so pain that is triggered by such a mechanism, for example stump and phantom limb pain, are often responsive to these drugs. They are also effective in diffuse burning-like pains often known by the term 'causalgia'.

Anxiolytic drugs

This group of drugs is sometimes employed for the treatment of chronic pain. The most commonly prescribed within the group are the benzodiazepines. These drugs are effective in relieving muscle spasm and are probably of some value in musculoskeletal strain or sprain. They are also very effective anxiolytics and anxiety associated with pain states should be relieved with these agents. A major problem with these drugs is their tendency to cause dependence and it is not recommended that they be prescribed for longer than two weeks at a time in most patients. This effectively restricts their use in chronic pain states although they may be of some value in patients who have episodic but infrequent muscle spasms. Even so, there is some doubt as to whether clinically significant relaxation of muscles is achieved even with high doses of these drugs.

A sedative drug called hydroxyzine is an interesting and rather surprising drug which is unrelated to the benzodiazepines and combines the properties of being anti-anxiety, anti-emetic and antihistamine (H_1 blocker). Although hydroxyzine potentiates the analgesic effects of opiates, no controlled trial has been carried out using this drug for chronic pain. It is, nevertheless, frequently used for this purpose in pain clinics, especially in the USA, where any effects that it produces may be due more to an anxiolytic action rather than to an analgesic mechanism.

Practical use of psychotropic drugs for the treatment of chronic pain

Antidepressants, antipsychotics, anticonvulsants and anti-anxiety drugs may be used in the control of chronic pain in order to produce one, or more, of the following effects:

1 analgesia

2 antidepressant action

3 hypnotic action

4 anti-anxiety effect

Examples of how drugs belonging to each of these four main groups are used for the relief of chronic pain will now be considered.

1   *Antidepressants*: Antidepressants are particularly valuable in the treatment of chronic headaches, facial pain, arthritic pain, post-herpetic neuralgia, cervical pain, low back pain, diabetic neuropathy and gastric ulcer. They are also considered to be effective in patients with terminal cancer pain although the evidence for their efficacy in this group of patients has not yet been established.

Tricyclic antidepressants are normally the drug of choice in these conditions, although there is a case for giving phenelzine or other MAOI drugs in facial pain. The tricyclics have a long half-life ($T\frac{1}{2}$) and it is therefore logical to prescribe them as a single daily dose to be taken at night so as to capitalise on their hypnotic effect. It is prudent to start therapy with a small dose, for example 25 mg at night for the first few days in order to check that the patient does not exibit intolerance to the drug. If the patient tolerates the drug well but requires a higher dose to control the pain (as is usually the case) then the dose can be *slowly* increased to 50–100 mg at night. Since these drugs have a long $T\frac{1}{2}$ (25–30 hours) it will take at least five times the half-life, i.e. 5–7 days to reach steady state after each change of dosage. (At steady state the amount of drug entering the body is just balanced by that leaving the body.) The patient should also be warned that the analgesic effect will not occur immediately but will take time to develop. It is sometimes helpful to measure the plasma concentration of the drug in order to ascertain that an adequate level has been reached or that compliance has been adequate. However, the precise level of drug in the blood that produces an analgesic effect is not known and these measurements can only be a guide to the most effective dosage. With drugs like phenelzine, it is usual to start with a dosage of 15 mg daily and then increase slowly by 15 mg at weekly or two-weekly intervals to a maximum of 60–70 mg daily. With the tricyclic drugs, analgesic effects often occur at a dosage of 75 mg *nocte*, although there is no contraindication to raising the dose up to a maximum of 150 mg *nocte* if there is no beneficial effect, provided that no unwanted effects ensue.

In general these antidepressants are well tolerated although potentially can produce a large spectrum of adverse effects. Their main unwanted effects are dry mouth, a feeling of light headedness and mild sedation. However, with the smaller range of dosage that is usually effective in producing relief of pain, this is less likely to be a problem. Medication can be continued for long periods without major adverse effects. With MAOIs such as phenelzine, it is vitally important that the patients avoid certain foods that are normally broken down by monoamine oxidase. If these foods are taken in the presence of an MAOI, a rapid rise of blood pressure can occur and deaths have been recorded. However, if the patient avoids food containing tyramine, the amine responsible for these effects, then this effect should be avoided. The foods concerned are cheese, certain red wines, meat extracts, pickled herring and game that has been hung for some time. The foods to avoid are normally listed on a card which is given to patients by the pharmacist at the time the drug is dispensed.

Experience with the newer antidepressants is not clearly established. However, low dosage incrementation as described for the other antidepressants is recommended. Little is known about the long-term use of these drugs.

2   *Antipsychotics*: It is rarely appropriate to use an antipsychotic drug as first choice in pain relief but it may be of some value as an adjunct to treatment with an antidepressant or anticonvulsant. The combination of perphenazine and amitriptyline in one tablet has been widely used although the evidence that this combination is more effective than either drug alone is lacking. Furthermore, combination tablets are relatively expensive and make it impossible to adjust the doses of each individual drug. It is better therefore to add perphenazine in a dosage of 2 mg to existing treatment and raise the dose to 6 mg maximum by four weeks if there has been no improvement at a lower dose. Fluphenazine or flupenthixol, both at a dosage of 0.5 mg, increasing to 1 mg daily are occasionally prescribed and at this low dose unwanted effects are rare.

This group of drugs can cause stiffness of the face and Parkinsonian movements. Although these unwanted effects can be overcome by anticholinergic drugs, it is not recommended that these be given to patients with chronic pain. In most cases the phenothiazine drugs should not be continued for long periods, although if unwanted effects are not present at a low dosage the drug can be continued.

Phenothiazines are known to precipitate or cause a movement disorder called tardive dyskinesia if given long term therefore continued use in patients with chronic pain is to be avoided.

3   *Anticonvulsants*: Anticonvulsant drugs are valuable in reducing pain when the cause of this is due to abnormal neuronal discharges from diseased or damaged nerves. They have been used for many years to treat trigeminal neuralgia and are also of value in phantom limb pains following amputation or after nerve damage from neuritis or other neuralgias.

Normally only one drug in this group is given at a time. The drug that is usually given first in these conditions is carbamazepine. This should be started in low dose and gradually increased. When the dosage reaches 500–600 mg per day some patients complain of unsteadiness on walking, dizziness, diarrhoea and nausea and vomiting. Occasional rashes can occur and aplastic anaemia has been reported very rarely. Patients who benefit from the drug are sometimes able to tolerate high doses. An average maintenance dose is of the order of 400–500 mg daily with a maximum of 1200 mg.

Another drug in the same group that is used in chronic pain states is sodium valproate. This drug is more rapidly eliminated than carbamazepine and needs to be given 2 or 3 times a day. There is some suggestion that patients who do not respond to carbamazepine may respond to sodium valproate. The drug has a similar spectrum of unwanted effects to carbamazepine although liver abnormalities can sometimes result from long term therapy. Phenytoin is now less often used.

4   *Anti-anxiety drugs*: Apart from hydroxyzine, these drugs should only be used rarely for chronic pain. Furthermore, there is no conclusive evidence that hydroxyzine is effective even though it is used. The new anxiety-reducing drug buspirone has not yet been evaluated in pain states.

If a benzodiazepine drug is used it should only be given for very short periods and for not longer than two weeks.

Examples of chronic pain conditions that can be treated by psychotropic drugs

1   Non-malignant Chronic Pain Conditions

Example: Post-herpetic neuralgia
Drugs:
First choice: start with amitriptyline 20 mg at night, slowly increasing to 75 mg at night. If necessary slowly increase further to 150 mg at night. If no pain relief occurs after 14–21 days on the maximum dosage then

Second choice: ADD sodium valproate 200 mg twice daily or thrice daily and try combination for 14 days.

If treatment is successful then continue treatment but every six months check liver function tests, carry out full blood count and *temporarily* withdraw drugs slowly to check that there is a continuing need for them.

Third choice: If combination of amitriptyline and sodium valproate ineffective then

consider carbamazepine in place of sodium valproate;

or

continue amitriptyline in the same dosage, stop sodium valproate, start fluphenazine 1 mg *nocte* and increase to 3 mg daily if necessary.

Example: Pain due to deafferentation,
         eg amputation stump pain;
             phantom limb pain;
             causalgia due to diabetic or other neuropathy.

Drugs:

First choice: carbamazepine 100 mg b.d. initially. Increase slowly up to total daily maximum of 1200 mg (if tolerated). Give trial for three weeks and check plasma concentration during third week $(5–10 \, mg/l = 21–42 \, \mu mol/l)$.

Second choice: phenytoin 100 mg b.d. initially. Increase slowly up to total daily maximum of 600 mg. Check plasma concentration during second week $(10–20 \, mg/l = 40–80 \, \mu mol/l)$.

Example: Central or thalamic pain

Drugs:

First choice: antidepressant
Second choice: antidepressant + anti-epileptic
Third choice: antidepressant + antipsychotic
Other choices: phenelzine (MAOI)
                or
                naloxone 4 mg i.v.
                or
                anticholinesterase
                or
                ?

2   Malignant Chronic Pain Conditions

Pain which is due to malignant disease is treated in the first place with conventional analgesics which include both non-steroidal anti-inflammatory drugs (NSAIDs) and also opiates (e.g. morphine) and opioids (methadone). Sometimes a combination of these drugs is used and the choice and dosage will depend both upon the cause of the

Table 8.2. Indications for Psychotropic Drugs in the Treatment of Chronic Pain and other symptoms due to Malignancy (Twycross and Lack, 1983)

Symptoms	Chlorpromazine	Diazepam	Amitriptyline
Insomnia	+	+ +	+
Depression			+ +
Overwhelming pain	+	+ +	
Anxiety	+	+ +	
Tension headaches	+	+ +	
Muscle spasm pain	+	+ +	
Nocturnal frequency			+ +
Nocturnal enuresis			+ +
Rectal 'tensemoid' pain	+ +	+	
Bladder 'tensemoid' pain	+ +	+	
Bladder spasm pain			+ +
Superficial dysaesthetic pain			+ +
Post-herpetic neuralgia			+ +

pain and the patient's response. It is only when the conventional analgesics fail to control certain symptoms that the addition of a psychotropic drug is indicated. Twycross and Lack (1983) have drawn up the indications for the use of three psychotropic drugs which can play a valuable part in the treatment of various symptoms which may accompany terminal cancer and which may not be controlled adequately by conventional analgesics (Table 8.2).

Summary

1 Selected psychotropic drugs, including antidepressants, anti-psychotic and anti-anxiety drugs, have been used increasingly in the management of chronic pain conditions since the 1950s.

2 These agents, alone or in combination, are used either as a primary analgesic or as a secondary analgesic (co-analgesic) in the treatment of certain intractable pain conditions that have usually failed to respond to other drugs (e.g. NSAIDs or opioids) or to other methods of pain relief.

3 Controlled clinical trials on the efficacy of psychotropic drugs for the relief of chronic pain are limited and relate mainly to the use of antidepressants.

4 The mechanisms of pain relief by psychotropics has yet to be fully elucidated but seem likely to be due to one or more of the following: (i) the modulation of certain neurotransmitters (e.g. noradrenaline, 5HT) where these are concerned with pain inhibitory systems in brain and spinal cord, (ii) altered emotional response to pain,

(iii) reduced anxiety, and (iv) reduced spontaneous firing of nerve impulse generators.

5 The analgesic action of these psychotropic drugs that are useful in the treatment of chronic pain appears to be separate from their other actions because the analgesic effect occurs: (i) more rapidly, and (ii) with a smaller dose than when the same drug is used for its psychotropic effect.

6 It may be concluded that selected psychotropic drugs used either alone or in combination with other drugs can play a valuable role in the treatment of some types of chronic pain. The choice of drug is largely empirical and the clinician must be prepared to change the drug and the dosage according to the response of the patient.

Acknowledgements

The authors wish to thank Dr Robert Twycross and Dr Sylvia Lack for permission to reproduce material collated from Tables 16.1 and 16.4 in *Symptom Control in Far Advanced Cancer: Pain Relief* (1983) published by Pitman, London.

They also wish to thank Mrs Margaret Cheek and Mrs Valerie Wright for excellent secretarial assistance.

References

Beaumont, G. and Seldrup, J. (1980) Comparative trial of clomipramine in the treatment of terminal pain. *Journal of International Medical Research,* **8** (Suppl. 3), 67

Budd, K. (1981) Non-analgesic drugs in the management of pain. In *Persistent Pain,* Vol. 3 (S. Lipton & J. Miles, Eds.) Academic Press, London, p. 223

Couch, J.R. and Hassanein, R.S. (1979) Amitriptyline in migraine prophylaxis. *Arch. Neurol.,* **36**, 695

Feinmann, C., Harris, M. and Cawley, R. (1984) Psychogenic facial pain: presentation and treatment. *British Medical Journal,* **288**, 436

Ganvir, P., Beaumont, G. and Seldrup, J. (1980) A comparative trial of clomipramine and placebo as adjunctive therapy in arthralgia. *J. Int. Med. Res.,* **8**, (Suppl. 3), 60

Gringras, M. (1976) A clinical trial of tofranil in rheumatic pain in general practice. *J. Int. Med. Res.,* **4** (Suppl. 2), 41

Hameroff, S. R., Randall, C. C., Scherer, K., Crago, B. R., Neuman, C., Womble, J. R. and Davis, T. P. (1982) Doxepin effects on chronic pain, depression and plasma opioids. *J. Clin. Psych.,* **43** (8), 22

Johansson, F. and Von Knorring, L. (1979) A double-blind controlled study of a serotonin uptake inhibitor (Zimelidine) versus placebo in chronic pain patients. *Pain,* **7**, 69

Lascelles, R.G. (1966) Atypical facial pain and depression. *British J. Psychiat.*, **112**, 651

Lance, J. W. and Curran, D. A. (1964) Treatment of chronic tension headache. *Lancet*, **1**, 1236

Lee, R. and Spencer, P. S. J. (1977) Antidepressants and pain: A review of the pharmacological data supporting the use of certain tricyclics in chronic pain. *J. Int. Med. Res.*, **5**, Suppl. (1), 146

McDonald Scott, W. A. (1969) The relief of pain with an antidepressant in arthritis. *Practitioner*, **202**, 802

MacNeill, A. L. and Dick, W. C. (1976) Imipramine and rheumatoid factor. *J. Int. Med. Res.*, **4** (Suppl. 2), 23

Merskey, H. (1977) Psychiatric Management of Patients with Chronic Pain. In 'Persistent Pain' vol. 1 (S. Lipton, Ed.) Academic Press, London, p. 113

Okasha, A., Ghalkeb, H. A. and Sadek, A. (1973) A double blind trial for the clinical management of psychogenic headache. *Br J. Psychiat.*, **122**, 181

Pilowsky, I., Hallett, B. C., Bassett, D. L., Thomas, P. G. and Penhall, R. K. (1982) A controlled study of amitriptyline in the treatment of chronic pain. *Pain*, **14**, 169

Sigwald, J., Herbert, H. and Quetin, A. (1957) The treatment of herpes and post-herpetic pain (and other resistant forms of pain) with phenothiazine derivatives. *Sem. Hop. Paris*, **33**, 1137

Twycross, R. G. and Lack, S. A. (1983) Symptom Control in Far Advanced Cancer: Pain Relief. Pitman, London

Walsh, T. D. (1983) Antidepressants in chronic pain. *Clin. Neuropharmacol.*, **6**, 271

Watson, C. P., Evans, R. J., Reed, K., Merskey, H., Goldsmith, L. and Warsh, J. (1982) Amitriptyline versus placebo in postherpetic neuralgia. *Neurology*, **32**, 671

9

Behavioural techniques

S. P. Tyrer

Introduction

Behavioural treatments are concerned with altering the behaviour of an individual. The principle on which behavioural techniques are based is that behaviour is directly related to its consequences. Actions that are followed by pleasurable experiences are more likely to be repeated whereas behaviours that are not rewarded or which have unpleasant consequences are likely to be reduced. This process is described as conditioning. The effects of conditioning can often have important implications for pain behaviour and these are reflected in at least two ways. The first is in relation to respondent or organic pain in which pain behaviour results from noxious stimuli that have occurred immediately previous to the onset of pain. In contrast, operant pain behaviour is that which occurs as a result of reward or relief of unpleasant symptoms. Assessment of pain behaviour involves the determination of how far each of these factors contributes to the presentation.

Behavioural assessment

The assessment of the patient with chronic pain has been described earlier (Chapter 7). However, particular factors which help to determine whether a patient is likely to need and respond to specific behavioural treatments may also be required. The aim of behavioural assessment is to identify pain behaviours, determine how far these are due to organic or operant causes and to assess which factors reinforce pain behaviour. As part of the more general assessment the mood state of the patient, the extent to which muscle tension plays a part in the genesis of pain and the assessment of stresses that contribute to pain complaint should also be obtained. It may be appropriate to use some of the instruments indicated in Chapter 7 for assessment of cognitive difficulties and coping strategies.

Behaviour in the outpatient clinic may not be representative of behaviour at home. A separate and joint interview with the spouse is essential to obtain a clear picture of behaviours that are exhibited during customary activities. The usual sequence of events is for the spouse to be seen briefly at the time of the first interview and the patient then completes a pain diary (*see* Appendix, page 201) and on the second visit the spouse is interviewed in more depth. Observations may be made subsequently of specific pain behaviours that occur frequently, to examine what situations or environmental stimuli immediately precede these and then to note the consequences that follow. It can never be assumed in advance which stimuli are reinforcers. For instance, social attention can be reinforcing to one person and yet unpleasant to another.

The assessment should be able to determine how far pain behaviour is governed by the consequences of that behaviour rather than physical nociceptive factors. Both of course may operate. However, before embarking on a behavioural programme, which takes up a good deal of therapist time, other treatments should be considered. If the effects of specific environmental factors contribute to the development of pain, attention should be specifically directed to the resolution of these. If these situations cannot be avoided, and this is usually the case, it may be appropriate to treat the anxiety arising from the feared situation by cognitive therapy, desensitisation or other procedures (*see* Chapter 11). If muscle tension contributes to the painful complaint, relaxation or hypnosis is likely to be a more appropriate treatment (*see* Chapters 10 and 12). Any of these treatments can be combined with a behavioural programme but the rationale for this should be set out at the start of treatment.

Treatment

The nature of the treatment selected will depend to a large extent on whether the patient is an inpatient or an outpatient. As most Pain Clinics do not have inpatient facilities an outpatient programme will be described first.

Outpatient programme

Treatment plan

At the very start it should be established that the patient wishes to lose his pain and that he is prepared to work hard at this. It must be made quite explicit that the Pain Clinic staff will help the patient toward this goal but that the patient himself is responsible for carrying out the actions that have been agreed between therapist and patient. If the patient assents to this and the therapist is confident about the motivation, an individualized plan indicating the aims of treatment, and how it is proposed that they should be achieved, should be agreed at the start of treatment. After discussion, realistic goals should be selected and measures discussed on how to achieve these. Exercises and procedures should also be identified that may help the patient in attaining the goal of pain reduction. Some clinics employ a written contract which has to be signed by both the patient and by the therapists. Whether such a contract is used or not there should be clear agreement between patient and staff about the aims of the treatment so that there is no misunderstanding. Complete elimination of pain is not normally a practical goal and this should be discussed to avoid misunderstanding. However, any programme should be flexible and should be tailored to the nature of the pain and abilities and progress of the patient.

The selection of appropriate goals to which the patient aspires is not always easy. In many cases, the patient says that he wishes to do a number of enjoyable things that he used to do before he developed his pain but in reality these may no longer be feasible because of the patient's physical handicap. However, it is a helpful opening question to ask the patient what he would do if his pain was reduced considerably. This will give some idea of what activities the patient previously enjoyed and what may be feasible in the future. The list of goals selected should not be confined to these; it is often valuable to choose any structured activity which employs the talents of the patient and which when completed leads to a sense of achievement. The goals selected should not just be in the physical domain; improvements should be sought in the area of emotional relationships if both patient and therapist think this is appropriate.

Some time will need to be spent on determining the most appropriate goals for each patient. These should also be agreed with the spouse or person with whom the patient is in daily close contact. However, a list of goals should be made out at every outpatient attendance where this has been decided beforehand; these can always be changed at the next interview if they are not thought to be achievable or as satisfying as the patient originally thought.

A typical selection of goals from a patient in the Newcastle Pain Relief Clinic is given below. The patient concerned was a 45-year-old man who had received a coronary artery bypass graft for severe cardiac ischaemia and who had continued to have the pain after the operation despite documented evidence of patent coronary arteries. He had given up his job as a fitter and spent virtually all his time at home with his wife, who also was becoming progressively more

Table 9.1. Targets in behavioural programme

Playing snooker

Week 1	Play once a week for 10 minutes
Week 2	Play twice a week for 10 minutes
Week 3	Play twice a week for 20 minutes
Week 4	Play twice a week for 30 minutes
Week 5	Play game all the way through.

Gardening

Week 1	Weed for 15 minutes
Week 2	Sow seeds for 20 minutes
Weeks 3–6	Gradually increase time doing varied tasks in garden.

Talk with wife

Week 1	Spend $\frac{1}{2}$ hour talking with wife at 7.30 p.m. on Friday
Week 5	Spent two $\frac{1}{2}$ hour intervals talking with wife each week.

physically ill with rheumatoid arthritis. The list of goals agreed with this patient are given below:

i   To play snooker two or three times a week at his local club.

ii To renovate his garden so that it would again grow vegetables throughout the year.

iii To talk more to wife about other matters than his and her health.

After the goals have been selected a plan is made which records the steps that will need to be completed to attain the overall goal. For instance, with the first target described above, it was agreed that the patient would go to his club and play a few balls on his own or with a friend for ten minutes only. It was then suggested that he sit back and watch a game or talk to some of the other players. This pattern was to be repeated on another occasion in the week and twice a week on subsequent weeks. A similar, relatively easily attained 'sub-goal' was selected for his gardening work. With regard to the third point a specific time was set aside each day, during and after the evening meal, when the couple would discuss matters of interest that they had come across in the day. Conversation about each other's health was to be avoided at this time. Succeeding steps in the programme are indicated in Table 9.1.

It is essential to discuss the selection of goals and sub-goals with both patient and spouse. In the patient described above he had found that before his operation that activity gave rise to chest pain and as similar pains occurred after the operation he assumed that his heart problem had recurred. Explanation that exercise in somebody who had been inactive and unfit can itself cause pain because of the lengthening of previously shortened muscle fibres, helped both the spouse and patient to acknowledge that the origin of his chest pain could be due to something other than a cardiac problem. The patient's wife was more accepting of this suggestion than her husband and on further visits it was clear that her supportive comments had encouraged him to attempt sub-goals that he might not have attempted otherwise.

The other reason for involving a spouse at all stages of treatment is to explain how attention by the spouse or others to complaint of pain by the sufferer may encourage pain behaviour. Instead of providing sympathetic involvement at these times the spouse should be advised to acknowledge that her partner has pain but not do anything that would reward him for his pain behaviour.

It is also important to explain the importance of the concept of 'pacing' at the time that the first sub-goal is chosen. Many patients, after weeks of inactivity, believe that they should go back to their old pursuits that they carried out before pain developed. They find that they feel exhausted after a short time and they often suffer pain for some hours and even days after the exercise because of the unaccustomed activity of their muscles. In the case described, a much less challenging sub-goal than that originally suggested had to be substituted because thirty minutes gardening gave rise to severe chest pain and considerable rumination. The patient and spouse should be told that pain levels are likely to increase during the first stages of treatment as unused muscles and joints are put into action. They should be encouraged to concentrate on the achievement in keeping to the sub-goals selected. When a number of these have been attained, the satisfaction in achievement helps to reduce the impact of the pain caused. As time goes on and muscle function improves the pain becomes less. However, it is very rare for the pain to be entirely abolished by a programme of this sort and in many cases there is only a slight improvement in pain ratings. But the improved function and consequent greater scope for occupation in more pleasurable pursuits counteracts this considerably. The improvement in function that occurs should constantly be stressed to the patient with reference to what they were doing before they started the programme.

The treatment plan is not confined to the goals selected. Other aspects of well behaviour should also be encouraged. The usual daily activities of living that have been avoided because of pain are broken down by the therapist into many small tasks. Going to town to shop would start with a walk around the local houses, then to a corner shop, then to town on a quiet day, and so on. At all times the therapist negotiates with the patient what is an achievable step as it is vital that the patient succeeds in these early stages. When setting targets for daily activity, the patient should be encouraged to generate most of the ideas himself. Activity should go ahead as much as possible within reasonable limits regardless of the pain level. All details of the intended stages should be discussed with the patient, i.e. when, with whom, how often, etc. and the therapist should anticipate as many problems as possible in advance. Success depends upon systematic and detailed behavioural tasks that are each met with some form of positive reinforcement, including self-praise, after successful achievement.

In patients who are reluctant to try out new activities because of their fear of making the pain worse, and in those where there is little support from others, supervised exercises by a physiotherapist should be arranged at the outpatient clinic. These are essential for less motivated clients in whom the evidence of extensive disability is strong. The physiotherapist observes the patient's posture, gait, range of movements and any deformities. After this assessment an exercise programme is normally selected and a homework assignment is given (*see* Chapter 15).

When somebody has pain and analgesic drugs are to hand it is usual to take these drugs when pain is at its most severe. The problem is that this practice encourages drug-taking when pain is proving a problem. If relief is obtained drug-taking is reinforced. This leads to an increase in the desire to take drugs in somebody who has persistent pain and as the opiate drugs in particular have the potential to cause dependence the sufferer may find himself rapidly increasing his drug intake. If administration of drugs is made non-contingent with pain, i.e. pain behaviour does not determine when the patient takes drugs this cycle can be broken. All drugs that are taken should be given according to the time on the clock, not because of increased pain. This avoids the possibilities of pain behaviour being reinforced by actual or perceived drug benefits. It may be appropriate to progressively withdraw analgesic medication, particularly if large doses of opiate drugs are being taken.

It is helpful to describe in some detail how this is brought about as gradual reduction in unnecessary medication is a common feature of many behavioural programmes although need not, of course, be confined to this mode of treatment.

Procedures in the withdrawal of analgesic medication

Analgesic drugs that act peripherally, as opposed to central action in the brain, are not difficult to withdraw and there are usually no major difficulties in doing this. However, with centrally acting drugs, particularly those that have any potential for causing dependence or addiction, it is essential to withdraw such agents slowly to avoid unpleasant withdrawal symptoms. In most patients with chronic pain the group of drugs to which this slow withdrawal schedule most frequently applies is the opiate drugs, which include a wide variety of agents from codeine to morphine. The benzodiazepine group of drugs

**Table 9.2. Equivalent dose of methadone compared to
other opiate drugs**

	Equivalent dose of methadone (mg/mg)
Morphine	100
Codeine	100
Dihydrocodeine	150
Pentazocine	600

are also sometimes prescribed in patients with chronic pain for the purpose of relaxing muscles, reducing anxiety or helping insomnia and the comments below apply to patients withdrawing from benzodiazepines, which may sometimes be antalgesic.

The simplest way of reducing any centrally acting drug is to diminish the dose by some 10% every few days and continue reduction until the drug is stopped. This may be a feasible course, and may be more successful with the benzodiazepines than with the opiates. However, many patients receiving opiates are psychologically and physically dependent upon them and if they know the dosage is gradually being withdrawn they complain of more severe symptoms. A frequent and effective way of achieving the same goal is to give the patient an equivalent amount of the opiate drug they are taking in a syrup vehicle and then gradually reduce the dosage of the active ingredients over time. This procedure of making up analgesic drugs in what is referred to as a 'pain cocktail', is widely used at our clinic and elsewhere and is often effective.

The principles are simple. An equivalent dose of an opioid drug that is readily miscible in water, such as methadone, is given to the patient in divided doses, three or four times a day. Table 9.2 indicates what the equivalent dosage of methadone is for some commonly prescribed opiate drugs.

The dosage and frequency of administration of the drug is noted in a special card in the Pain Clinic and the patient obtains his pain cocktail from the pharmacy. The patient is told that the dosage of drug in the pain cocktail will be adjusted according to his needs but invariably this is downward, although it is permissible to maintain an identical dosage if pain intensity increases considerably. However, in most cases this is not necessary and it is heartening to find how many patients improve both in terms of their well-being and severity of pain as the dosage of opiates is gradually withdrawn. On successive visits to the clinic the same quantity of fruit-flavoured vehicle is prescribed but the dosage of methadone is gradually reduced by some 10% every month or six weeks. Sufficient drug is given to last until the next appointment and other doctors involved in the patient's care should be asked not to prescribe any other analgesic medication while they are on the pain cocktail. Once the patient reaches the stage where there is no active ingredient in the pain cocktail it is usual to continue the unadulterated fruit syrup for a further month or so and then gradually withdraw this. Most patients are quite content with this procedure and accept the doctor's instructions. If the patient asks, the therapist should be frank and inform the patient that there is no active ingredient in the mixture when this is the case.

Haloperidol and clonidine have also been used in helping patients to withdraw from opioids. The success of these drugs is much more likely when used in an inpatient setting.

Monitoring of progress

The patient should be seen at frequent intervals after the first consultation. If the spouse is also able to attend this is of considerable advantage. If possible, visits should be arranged at weekly or two-weekly intervals to begin with and once gains have been made at longer intervals thereafter. In addition to recording success or otherwise in reaching the sub-goals (Table 9.1) it is also valuable for the patient to complete a diary of activities at regular intervals. The pain diary illustrated on page 201 can be completed. In patients who spend a good deal of time lying down during the day a more focused diary should be selected.

In all types of human endeavour carefully thought out plans do not always come to fruition. 'The best laid schemes o' mice an' men gang aft a'gley'. Robert Burn's words are as apt now as they were when they were written 200 years ago. For a variety of reasons during a behavioural programme there will be times when achievements laboriously garnered over a number of weeks appear to be irrevocably lost in the patient's eyes and he feels like giving up altogether. It is vital to recognize that these periods often occur but they can be solved if an appropriate strategy is developed to deal with them. A written plan is formulated specifying what changes should be made to the programme and when these should be implemented. Usually, the reason for patients discontinuing behavioural programmes is because of an increase in pain. If pain does increase by more than an agreed amount from baseline (often expressed as a persistent score of over 9 on the 10 cm pain line) and the patient wishes to ease off the behavioural programme for a time, the plan is put into effect. It is vital that the patient informs his or her spouse or other person close to them at this time. It may also be advisable to contact the therapist, although this depends to a large extent on the assessment of the judgement and resources of the patient and spouse.

Once a decision has been made to suspend the programme a new, short behavioural plan is started. This should be adjusted according to the needs of the patients but usually involves increase in rest time, decrease in activity and increase in distracting coping strategies such as playing board games, writing. It is understood that this new temporary programme will be time-limited and after two or three days the patient will return to the old programme.

If there are frequent breaks of this nature in the behavioural programme the original plan may need to be revised.

Once function is improved patients become more confident and should be encouraged to develop their own further goals for subsequent treatment. As the patients become more optimistic they are seen less regularly although it is a good idea to maintain contact for up to two years after the programme is started. We often encourage patients to keep in touch by letter. If this is not received by the expected date it is advisable to get in touch with the patient directly. Patients may have attended a pain education class (*see* Chapter 13) and, once these have been completed, patients may continue to meet. These groups can be valuable in providing support for others with similar pain problems.

Inpatient programme

Treatment programme

Inpatient treatment is required for patients who live far away from outpatient centres, for patients in whom illness behaviour has been encouraged by the spouse or close companion and for many patients who have a severe disability, e.g. wheelchair-bound. It may also be required for patients who fail to respond to an outpatient programme although it is important to consider the reasons for failure before automatically including such patients for inpatient treatment. Above all, the motivation of the patient to cooperate with treatment should be paramount. The two inpatient units in the United Kingdom, in Glasgow and London, that are involved in inpatient treatment have broadly similar formats which are to a large extent derived from programmes in the United States of America and Canada. Experience of those involved in these programmes strongly suggests that inpatient facilities should be based on rehabilitation principles and there may be advantages in having the unit attached to physical rehabilitation facilities. It is not advisable to have such inpatient programmes attached to psychiatric units.

Patients are normally admitted to an inpatient unit in groups of four to six for a defined period of time of four to six weeks. There are advantages in having a new group of patients admitted halfway through the programme so that the learning of the procedures involved can be facilitated. After baseline assessments of pain, activity and mood a structured programme is started with activities or talks scheduled throughout the day. The emphasis is on increasing well behaviours, particularly physical activity, and reducing pain behaviours. Daily targets are set for activities such as walking, climbing stairs and the number of 'sit-ups' from a reclining position, gradually increasing over time.

In between the frequent exercises and activities, patients are taught how to relax and there are regular education sessions on the causes of pain and the part that physical and psychological factors play in this. Most patients attending such units have been receiving drugs for long periods with little positive effect and reduction of these is often beneficial. Again, a regular daily reduction in drug intake is usually implemented shortly after admission to the unit.

Although much of the day is spent with other patients in groups, individual attention is given at least once a day to each patient. All activities, medication reduction and mood are regularly assessed and there is constant feedback to the patient to help encourage him. Each patient carries their own personal diary around with them at all times and as targets are achieved they are recorded. Increase in time spent at a task is helped by the use of timing devices which issue a bleep once the required time has been spent on the activity in question. This also ensures that patients do not do more than they should too early in the programme.

As far as possible, spouses or living companions are involved in individual discussions with the patient about their progress. A useful time for these discussions is at the end of the week before the patient goes home for the weekend. Many inpatient programmes are closed at weekends which reduces running costs considerably. Before the patient is discharged from the clinic it is vital to involve the spouse in designing an outpatient behavioural programme as described earlier in this chapter.

Contraindications to behavioural treatment

Behavioural programmes are expensive and only those patients who need these should be selected for treatment. If the patient is reasonably independent and resourceful despite their pain a behavioural programme may not need to be intensively carried out although the principles of treatment are still a mainstay of success. On the other hand, there are some patients who are so locked in to a lifestyle with a spouse for whom the patient's pain behaviour has positive assets. In such cases any form of programme designed to reduce pain behaviour is unlikely to succeed and such patients should not be selected. The evidence of poor motivation may only become apparent once a programme is started but if there is poor compliance early on with the targets that have been agreed between patient and therapist and this is not due to misunderstanding or selecting targets that are difficult to achieve, the continued inclusion of the patient in the programme should be reassessed. It has been found that patients who are involved in a compensation claim do not do well in behavioural programmes until after their claim has been settled.

Those operating behavioural programmes should be flexible in the design of these. During the early stages of these programmes it may become apparent that particular stresses are associated with an increase in pain or that there is considerable reluctance by the patient to carry out manoeuvres that are recommended by the therapist. In such cases it is necessary to explain in detail to the patient exactly what factors are contributing to the pain and it may be necessary to use biofeedback procedures to illustrate to the patient how stress and apprehension can cause muscle tension and muscle pain. In these patients, relaxation procedures should be combined with the behavioural measures. There are some advantages in such patients being admitted to inpatient units as patients who are concerned that their pain represents evidence of tissue damage and have thought this for many years find it difficult to initiate any activity that causes pain unless carefully and consistently cajoled to do so. This is often more feasible in an inpatient unit.

Summary

Although the principles of behaviour therapy should be used by all professionals involved with the chronic pain patient, specific behavioural treatment programmes should normally only be given to patients whose pain behaviour has been encouraged directly or indirectly by others, and where there is no evidence of sufficient organic pathology to account for the degree of pain behaviour exhibited. In most cases, as long as the patient does not have a great distance to travel, outpatient programmes are effective if the patient and spouse are motivated. A treatment plan is drawn up with the agreement of both patient and therapist that includes selected targets for which to aim, and goals identified necessary for attaining these. At the same time as improvements in function are occurring medication is normally reduced, unless it is absolutely necessary, and other everyday activities in which the patient used to be employed are encouraged by setting further behavioural targets.

Inpatient programmes may be necessary for those patients who live too far away from major centres, where there is extensive disability, and where there is poor spouse motivation. The same principles apply as for an outpatient programme but the programme is much more intensive, being completed within a matter of a few weeks. It is often necessary to involve other procedures such as relaxation and stress avoidance techniques during behavioural programmes. Flexibility of approach should be the watchword.

Bibliography

Gil, K. M., Ross, S. L. and Keefe, F. J. (1988) Behavioral treatment of chronic pain: four pain management protocols. *Chronic Pain*, **19**, 377–413

Keefe, F. J., Crisson, J. E. and Snipes, M. T. (1986) Observational methods for assessing pain: a practical guide. In *Applications in Behavioral Medicine and Health Psychology: A Clinician's Sourcebook* (eds J. A. Blumenthal, and D. C. McKee), Sarasota, Florida, Professional Resource Exchange

10

Use of relaxation

P. T. James

Introduction

Outside sleep, three aspects of bodily functioning can be discerned which are relevant to chronic pain and amenable to relaxation therapy.

1 Cortical arousal (alertness of the brain)

2 Sympathetic nervous system activation

3 Muscle tension

Arousal, activation and muscle tension are closely related and if there is an increase in degree of stimulation of one system this tends to affect the others.

Cortical Arousal

The term 'cortical arousal' refers to the degree of alertness of the brain. When we are aroused by events occurring in our close environment, there is increased activity of the cerebral cortex. This is associated with an increase of emotional intensity, e.g. anxiety, anger, excitement or elation. Worrying thoughts will be more preoccupying and distressing with increased arousal. This can contribute to the development of insomnia.

Sympathetic Activation

The sympathetic nervous system, part of the autonomic or self-regulating system, normally prompts us for action. It is sometimes called the 'fight and flight' system as it is brought into action when we are faced by threats that we advance to face or from which we run away. When challenged by such dangers there is an increase in heart rate and amount of blood pumped out by the heart, more rapid respiration, increased temperature and sweating. These changes are brought about by both an increase in (sympathetic) nervous system activity and by release of hormones into the blood from the pituitary and adrenal glands.

These same effects are brought about by stress. Stress can be defined in different ways but essentially involves a bodily reaction to perceived threats in the environment, and whether this occurs or not depends on the personality of the person exposed and his previous life experiences. The physical and mental consequences of stress accumulate over time. In those exposed to stress of this nature these physical feelings may be misinterpreted as symptoms of illness.

Chronic pain is a potent stressor. In addition to the symptoms described, relatives may notice increased irritability or emotionality. A minority will experience panic attacks at these times which may further increase emotionality and physical disability.

Muscle tension

In the voluntary striated muscles of the body, i.e. those concerned with voluntary movement, there are background levels of activity which maintain body posture. Increased activity in these muscles can result because of bad posture, using guarding manoeuvres in a mistaken attempt to reduce pain, and through anxiety or stress. Prolonged muscle tension is associated with an increase in both sympathetic activation and cortical arousal.

Rationale of relaxation therapy

Conditions where muscle tension directly influences the neuronal activity of peripheral pain pathways will be particularly suited to muscle relaxation therapy (e.g. myofascial pain). The specific muscle groups involved in the condition may be targeted for muscle relaxation or biofeedback. However, many other conditions occur where over-arousal and increased sympathetic tone may also respond to relaxation. The gate control model of pain predicts that reduction of muscle tension in any pain condition, even when there is no muscle related aetiology, will reduce pain sensation. Pain itself is a major stressor, and so often leads to an increase in muscle tension generally. Thus, an individual may adopt a body stance to try and guard against the pain getting worse; this increases muscle tension in associated muscle groups and itself increases pain. Such pain-induced tension can become quite automatic leading to a vicious cycle causing more pain. Relaxation at times of increased stress is particularly valuable in this regard. Teaching muscle relaxation can also be directly aimed at maintaining a better posture. Throughout the therapist is encouraging the individual to maintain muscle levels at a lower and more relaxed level whilst still engaging in daily activities.

Emotions such as anxiety, perhaps described as stress by some, can directly increase pain sensation levels, and reduce pain tolerance. Furthermore, an important dimension of chronic pain is the associated distress or pain affect on the quality of life and pain behaviour. These emotions are directly magnified by arousal and activation. Therefore, relaxation methods which reduce arousal and activation can reduce pain affect, and possible pain sensation levels. This is especially true for people who are prone to strong emotions because of their constitutional vulnerability, their recent life events, or current stressors/problems, or because of their belief of threat and loss resulting from the pain condition (*see* Chapter 3). For these individuals reducing arousal and activation is more important than simply lowering muscle tension.

Relaxation procedures involve a reduction in attention on anxiety-provoking thoughts. The most direct way of inducing mental calm is by occupying the mind on something neutral and unstimulating. If attention is occupied in this way, then it is necessarily being diverted away from the pain. hence relaxation may be a useful distraction method. Such distraction may be particularly useful when external stimuli are less evident, for example at night or when the individual is alone. A specific relaxation method should be selected at this time. It may be best directed by an external stimulus, such as a voice on a tape. A choice or a combination of different relaxation methods may also help the individual to attend without becoming too bored, and therefore, inattentive.

Learning a relaxation method can help an individual to gain a sense of control over their condition. There is some evidence that with increased perceived control, pain tolerance can be raised. It can also be a first step in encouraging individuals to take a greater responsibility for the self-management of their own condition. Whatever the approach used, the teaching should be thorough and broken into small steps to help overcome any learned helplessness.

Providing that a sufficiently persuasive rationale for the relaxation can be found and expectations of a good outcome are high, then patients may improve because of their expectations of improvement. This short-term benefit may initiate a more constructive pain evaluation and reduce pain affect, as well as increasing well behaviour. Progressive muscle relaxation is a concrete approach which treats the individual's pain in physical ways, and so is often more accepting to the patient. It is also the technique over which the therapist has most control early in treatment.

Relaxation training guidelines

The rationale for using a particular method needs to be tailored to the individual. An example below shows how the therapist attempts to negotiate the approach:

> From your pain diary you seemed to find that your pain gets worse when you get uptight or stressed, would you agree? If you learnt a relaxation skill you could keep yourself calmer. This would stop the pain getting worse at times of stress. Does that make sense to you? It may be worth trying a relaxation method. Do you notice much tension in your muscles? (patient acknowledges this). Shall we start with relaxing them?'

Once the therapist has a tentative agreement about the underlying rationale, he or she can extend this with analogies, demonstrations, and case examples. Throughout training clients are given every opportunity to express their doubts or concerns about the approach used.

Next the therapist needs to ensure that the pain patient has realistic expectations. Often people give up relaxation therapy prematurely because it did not work during the first week, it did not completely take the pain away, or because it had no effect when the pain was particularly bad. In fact as with any skill time is needed to acquire it.

For all relaxation methods an audio tape should ideally be made with instructions. However, all too often this prerecorded audio tape is all that patients receive. Although a useful adjunct to relaxation therapy it is not sufficient. It fails to tailor the method to the individual, it does not check for misunderstanding, it does not help motivate the patient, and it is not the best method of teaching a new skill. New skills are best learnt by modelling what is required with ample practice and feedback (especially praise) about performance. The therapist will also need to specify in detail what homework or practice is required between sessions, and review difficulties.

When teaching relaxation, attention is focused on bodily sensations. The therapist needs to ensure that individuals are not becoming too preoccupied with these as this can encourage introspection about pain sensation and related anxiety. To reduce this risk other bodily sensations can be emphasized, or less time can be spent on relaxation exercises by using relaxation *responses* (*see* p. 128). In a small number of cases relaxation may need to be temporarily stopped to allow clients to express anxiety-provoking thoughts which the training has engendered.

The physical setting in which relaxation procedures are carried out should have specific characteristics. The room should be quiet with dim lighting and have a chair with head support or bed with several pillows to enable the subject to sit, and be at a comfortable temperature. The patient should have used the toilet beforehand if necessary, and have undone tight clothing. Sufficient time, at least 30 minutes, should be allocated for the exercise. After the procedure there should be a minute or two to enable the patient to gradually readjust; sudden movement after relaxation is definitely contra-indicated.

When pain levels are high it is difficult for the subject to concentrate on the exercise. Consequently success with relaxation is unlikely, and this can be disillusioning if the subject's expectations are unrealistic. It is important to practice relaxation when the pain is less severe for two or three months until skills have been acquired.

Once the chronic pain patient has relaxation skills in the form of exercises, lasting more than ten minutes, and relaxation responses, lasting seconds, to manage their pain, they then have a choice on how best to use them. Although the exercises can be used routinely at certain times, they can be used as a strategy when pain levels begin to increase, when tension or anxiety is noted, or when distraction is required. The relaxation *responses* are particularly useful to keep tension levels down whilst engaging in well behaviour, or when being provoked by stressful situations or worrying thoughts. They can be used to reverse the subtle but detectable increases in activation, arousal and muscle tension associated with everyday hassles that would have been ignored before chronic pain developed.

If an individual has had pain for a long time, and has tried many therapies, some time may need to be spent to convince him that relaxation therapy is worth trying. Exercises should be carefully graded to avoid overloading people whose confidence is often at a low ebb.

Relaxation methods

Breathing Exercises

Slow and steady breathing is a relatively simple procedure to learn, and the effects on activation are quickly discernible. With the patient sitting or lying comfortably, arms on their lap, and eyes closed, the therapist first draws attention to the breathing cycle. It is explained that this can be consciously controlled to bring about a general calming, and that conversely breathing becomes irregular and rapid with tension. With the patient's eyes open the therapist demonstrates a succession of breathing cycles. He fills his lungs slowly by inhalation via the nose to a slightly exaggerated capacity, counting from 1 to 3 during the process. He then exhales even more slowly at a steady rate, counting throughout. This should not be so slow that breathlessness is caused.

The therapist then asks the patient to follow instructions, counting during inhalation and exhalation for a few minutes, subsequently enquiring about the comfort of this procedure. The breathing exercises can then be extended for longer periods. A number of variations exist which can be selected for different pain problems and separate patient characteristics.

1 The patient is encouraged to extend the exhalation even further without causing breathlessness.

2 The patient can exhale through parted lips, and imagine he is breathing over a candle he must not extinguish.

3 As the patient breathes in, he should be encouraged to take note of the tension in the chest walls, and then notice the relaxation and easement as he breathes out. Relaxation of the chest wall muscles is itself generalized to other muscles of the body.

4 As the patient breathes out he can say to himself words implying relaxation, e.g. 'calming', 'peaceful'.

5 Imagery can be used to construe inhalation as producing energy which on exhalation can be directed with good effect at the site of pain.

6 Abdominal breathing, in which the diaphragm ascends and descends during breathing, may be helpful.

The patient may be given an audio tape at the start with breathing cycles already counted, but this can usually be dispensed with. The patient should be encouraged to use breathing cycles throughout their daily activities.

Progressive and differential muscle relaxation

This was one of the earliest methods of relaxation developed by Jacobsen, but adapted over time (Bernstein and Borkovec, 1983). The primary aim is to concentrate specifically upon the relaxing of striate (voluntary) muscles throughout the body. One technique involves tension-release exercises which are designed to leave the muscles more relaxed, known as active muscle relaxation (*see* Table 10.1 and Appendix to this chapter). Alternatively, the muscles can be allowed to relax simply by consciously allowing and willing this to happen, for these muscles are under voluntary control. This is described as passive muscle relaxation (p. 134). Usually active muscle relaxation is preferred because the contrast between tension and relaxation is a useful distinction to learn. However, where tensing muscles actually causes severe pain, e.g. arthritis, or where tensing muscles is not followed by a subsequent relaxation, passive muscle relaxation should be the preferred method. Clinicians can of course combine the approaches for a given individual, initiating active relaxation for some muscle groups of the body with passive relaxation for the remainder.

Differential muscle relaxation simply refers to the skill of relaxing some muscle groups whilst others remain unchanged. This is a particularly useful goal in chronic pain for two reasons. Firstly, some tense muscle groups may be directly associated with pain, and so can be targeted specifically for relaxation. Secondly, to achieve significant changes in pain, the individual needs to continually relax some muscles throughout the day, while others are tense through use. Differential muscle relaxation is clearly consistent with this.

To begin with, inducing muscle relaxation may take 20 or 30 minutes in a quiet undisturbed room. However, subsequently the subject can usually be trained to relax very quickly in a matter of seconds. Training is directed to teaching the patient about quick muscle relaxation, following a cue. A cue is any voluntary action or environmental situation that is usually followed by a feeling of relaxation. Commonly used cues are words such as 'calm', 'relax' and 'ease' to bring about a quick coordinated relaxation of muscles. This is only possible after practising for some time.

Instructions for muscle relaxation

The subject sits in a comfortable armchair with head supported, or lies on a bed or couch, with eyes closed. The therapist explains that muscles are under our own control, and that as with any other skill we can learn to relax them more effectively if we practice. The rationale of the treatment is explained and the effects on the subject's pain is discussed and predicted.

Active Muscle Relaxation

A series of muscle groups are identified (Table 10.1) and subjected to tension-release cycles in sequence. Attention is first drawn to the sensation coming from each muscle group. Then for approximately six seconds, muscle tension is created in the selected muscle group, followed by a 20–30 second relaxation period. This tension-release cycle is repeated a second time. It is advisable for the therapist to rehearse the tension-release exercises in advance to ensure that this does not greatly increase the pain, and to ensure that the subject knows what is expected of him/her. Where cramp might be suspected, particularly in clients with poorer circulation to the legs, the muscle groups can be tensed less vigorously or for a shorter period. According to the underlying rationale, this should be sufficient to enable the muscles to start to relax and allow the individual to learn the contrast. Other muscle groups are then selected (Table 10.1). When all the muscles have undergone the tension-release exercises the subject spends another minute or so allowing the muscles to relax more fully each time they breathe out. Typical instructions are:

Table 10.1. Sequence of muscle groups

Muscle group	Typical signs of tension	To increase tension	In relaxation
Left arm or hand	Clenching of fist, arms crossed	Fist tight, arm straight and pulled into body	Fist open, arm supported on lap, arm heavy
Right arm or hand	Clenching of fist, arms crossed	Fist tight, arm straight and pulled into body	Fist open, arm supported on lap, arm heavy
Forehead and eyes	Frowning, often when concentrating	Eyes tightly shut, forehead screwed up	Forehead clear and even, eyes gently closed
Jaw and mouth	Grinding or tense jaw, lips tightly closed	Jaws tightly shut, cheeks pulled in and lips pressed together	Jaws apart, mouth slightly open
Neck	Tight and painful, especially at back	Push head backward onto chair or bed and yet attempt to pull head forward at same time	Head evenly and loosely supported by neck, neck muscles
Shoulders and back	Shoulders forward or up in the air, pressure across back. Back curved	Put shoulders back into bed or chair	Shoulders drawn and to sides. Shoulders and back pressing heavily against support. Back straight
Stomach	Holding muscles in stomach	Pull in stomach by tensing muscles	Let stomach out by relaxing muscles
Left leg	Crossed legs, sitting forward in chair	First pointed away, leg straight and pulled upwards into body	Leg heavy, no muscles pulling against each other
Right leg	Crossed legs, sitting forward in chair	First pointed away, leg straight and pulled upwards into body	Leg heavy, no muscles pulling against each other

'Concentrate as best you can on the sensations in your (named muscle group), notice what they are like when I say '*Now*, increase the tension by... (procedure in Table 10.1), build up the tension *Now*, 1, notice the tension, 2 and 3, building up tension, 4, feel the muscles pull, 5, notice what it's like 'hold on tight', 6, Okay and now *Relax*, let the tension go from your (named muscle group)'. The therapist continually asks the subjects to become more aware of the contrast between tension and relaxation, encourages them to look for sensations compatible with relaxation (e.g. heaviness) and invites them to gently return their attention to the exercises when they are inevitably distracted. It is good and more effective practice for the therapist to demonstrate and rehearse muscle relaxation for the patient in person rather than providing a pre-recorded tape. The therapist can take pain ratings before and after the exercise; the level will often be lower at the end and hence reinforce the procedure. The exercise will often reveal some muscle groups which are difficult to relax, and these then become the subject of more exercises. A full description of an active muscle relaxation session is given in the Appendix to this chapter.

Passive Muscle Relaxation

Passive muscle relaxation follows the same procedural sequence but without increasing muscle tension. The therapist has a more important role in verbally encouraging the subject to relax targeted muscles, especially by suggesting the sort of sensations that might be expected. Some of the simpler suggestions can be added to give a list of comments made initially by the therapist, but later by the subjects themselves. Repetition is an integral component.

Suggestions/Comments

Notice what the muscles are like (therapist name, as listed in Table 10.1).

You can change the muscle tension in your....

Notice the change as the muscles relax

Looking for (specify general expectations from Table 10.1)

Heavier and more relaxed

Your (body part) is becoming heavier and warmer

Your (body part) is letting go, relaxing, letting go

Your breathing is becoming slower and more regular

An example of passive relaxation is shown in the Appendix to this chapter. As the subject takes over control of the exercises the 'you' is substituted by 'I'.

Meditation

We know that a person's internal thinking can be quite anxiety or tension provoking, whereas distracting attention to pleasant and calming events, memories or plans can be relaxing. In Chapter 11 the use of imagery to relax and occupy the mind is described. However, an alternative to distraction by something positive, is to occupy attention by something quite meaningless and essentially unstimulating. This is the basic component of a variety of meditational techniques such as transcendental meditation, yoga, or t' ai chi. The task in meditation is to focus attention on what is called a 'mantra', which can be anything from a word to the air expelled from the nose during breathing. The novice meditator will need guidance to clear all but the mantra from the mind.

As with other relaxation methods, initial training benefits from a quiet and undisturbed environment, but with expert use the meditator can use this method almost anywhere. The subject closes his eyes and relaxes by physical methods (breathing and muscles) for a minute or two. He then gently focuses his attention upon his chosen mantra. As other thoughts immediately enter, these are let go in favour of the mantra. Meditators are encouraged to enjoy the process of letting go of their thoughts in favour of the mantra. Specifically, the 'forcing' of non-mantra thoughts away is discouraged. The following are suggestions for a mantra:

Saying 'one' on breathing out

Uttering meaningless three-syllable words, e.g. 'um-ban-ta', 'ay-eem-ra'

Concentrating on the sensation on the upper lip on breathing out through your nose

Focusing on the warmth of the stomach

There is no evidence to suggest that one mantra is better than another.

Each meditation session can take between 15 and 30 minutes. Meditating for longer periods, such as an hour or more, may be associated with unpleasant/unusual sensations and is not advised. Two meditation periods a day are usually recommended, and at least once a day is necessary for the novice to acquire this difficult skill.

Relaxation responses

Prolonged relaxation exercises lead to deep relaxation and such low levels of arousal that sleep may easily ensue. However, the primary aim of this treatment is to reduce activation and muscle tension throughout the day, especially to prevent escalating muscle tension produced by daily activities. To achieve this a quick 'calming', or 'quietening' response is required which still leaves the individual alert. One way is cued relaxation, a variant of progressive muscle relaxation noted earlier. This is also known as a relaxation response.

An example of a relaxation response involves one breathing cycle. The subject says a cue to himself such as 'calmer and easier' and takes in a slow deliberate but not too deep breath to a count of three. Simultaneously the individual scans their muscles (Table 10.1), to look for tension. This is followed by a slower, deliberate steady breath out whilst counting four coupled with relaxation of the identified tense muscles. A sensation of warmth is usually noticed in the stomach at this stage and is allowed to spread according to the wishes of the individual. This technique can be used literally hundreds of times a day and with regular practice can become an automatic response which does not have to be consciously controlled.

Other relaxation responses use imagery of previously experienced relaxing situations such as sitting in a summer house on a warm August day or listening to a known tranquil piece of music. It is worth asking the subject to identify details of past occasions when relaxation has occurred.

Biofeedback

Biofeedback refers to any technique that conveys physiological data that derives from the subject back to the subject concerned. At its simplest level, a measure such as the subject's heart beat can be amplified to produce a sound, or alternatively it can be averaged and displayed visually. Biofeedback is used to help people gain control of their physiological state and is commonly used to inform subjects when they are under stress. This may be identified and measured in different ways, e.g. muscle tension by electromyogram (EMG), sympathetic activation by heart rate or skin conductance, or arousal by electroencephalogram (EEG).

The most plausible use of biofeedback is for muscle relaxation by EMG feedback of specific muscle groups. The muscles in the head and neck and the paraspinal muscles are often under tension in localized painful states. It is relatively simple to place electrodes, record a baseline, and conduct biofeedback sessions with auditory feedback indicating average levels of muscle tension, perhaps in several muscle groups simultaneously. Patients are encouraged to reduce muscle tension in whatever way they can and this is then reinforced by a change in auditory feedback.

Twelve weekly sessions of one hour's duration is a typical course, though it can be more intense. One or two sessions may be used to illustrate how muscle tension causes pain. Suitable equipment for EMG biofeedback is quite expensive, but can provide a useful alternative to other methods. It can of course be combined with other techniques such as progressive muscle relaxation.

Therapists need to ensure that with the use of biofeedback they are not taking the responsibility for management away from the individual. All too often the patient is not acknowledging an active role, and is happy for the professional to do things to him. However, non-psychologically-minded individuals may accept the practical nature of biofeedback, and hence be engaged whilst other broader approaches are attempted. In some cases the clear relationship between the experience of pain and biofeedback measures and the effect of self-initiated techniques in controlling both of these can be very reinforcing, and may provide motivation for the patient who was originally sceptical of the value of his active intervention.

The rationale for biofeedback is that the information received by the subject will enable him to learn to control those physiological systems being monitored. However, apart from reducing muscle tension, most subjects are not able to alter easily these physiological measures. Most studies comparing biofeedback with muscle relaxation methods show the latter to be equally effective at first, and more effective when compared after treatment has been completed. It appears that biofeedback is not particularly successful at teaching new skills, but is useful within a session to reduce activation and arousal. Unless patients are unable or reluctant to use other techniques and biofeedback impresses them by its technology, other relaxation methods should normally be preferred.

Choice of relaxation methods

The methods of relaxation described in this chapter have generally been found to be of equal efficacy in controlled studies. The subject's choice, therefore, is of particular importance in selecting treatment. The more training and guidance that is given, the better the response. Particular attention should be paid to relaxation training during acute episodes of pain. The techniques for overcoming these are difficult to learn but subjects can be trained with sufficient education and practice. Even if pain sensation levels do not change much, there is good reason to expect an improvement in the quality of life.

Bibliography

Bernstein, D. A. and Borkovec, T. D. (1983) *Progressive Muscle Relaxation.* Research Press, Champaign, Ill.

Broome, A. and Jellicoe, H. (1987) *Living with Pain*. British Psychological Society/Methuen, Leicester

Catalano, E. M. (1987) *The Chronic Pain Control Workbook*. New Harbinger Publications Inc., Oakland, Calif.

Holzman, A. D. and Turk, D. C. (1986) *Pain Management: A Handbook of Psychological Treatment Approaches*. Pergamon Press, New York

Luthe, W. and Schultz, J. H. (1969) *Autogenic Therapy*. Grune and Stratton, New York

Poppen R. (1988) *Behavioural Relaxation Training and Assessment*. Pergamon Press, New York

Shapiro, D. H. and Walsh, R. N. (1984) *Meditation: Classic and Contemporary Perspectives*. Aldine, New York

Appendix

Active Muscle Relaxation

Settle back as comfortably as you can, let yourself relax to the best of your ability. Close your eyes, relax your arms by your sides, put your legs straight out in front of you. I now want you to concentrate on various parts of your body in turn. First I want you to concentrate on your right hand. Breathe deeply in and out. Now as you relax, clench your right fist, just clench your fist tighter and tighter and study the tension as you do so. Keep it clenched and feel the tension in your right fist and arm...and now relax...let the fingers of your right hand become loose and observe the contrast in your feelings. Now let yourself go and try to become relaxed all over. Once more clench your right fist really tight, hold it and notice the tension again. Now let go...relax. Let your fingers straighten out and notice the difference once more. Now repeat that with your left fist. Clench your left fist while the rest of your body relaxes. Clench that fist tighter and feel the tension...tenser and tenser...and now relax. Again enjoy the contrast. Repeat once more, clench the left fist, tight and tense, tense and tight...and now do the opposite of tension, relax and feel the difference. Continuing relaxing like that for a while. Relax your hands and forearms more and more. Now bend your elbows and tense your biceps muscles. Tense them harder and study the tension feelings. Now straighten out your arms, let them relax and feel that difference again. Let the relaxation develop. Once more tense your biceps, hold the tension and observe it carefully...now straighten the arms and relax. Each time you do this pay close attention to your feelings when you tense up and when you relax. Now straighten your arms, straighten them so that you feel most tension in the triceps muscles. (The triceps muscle is the muscle along the back of your upper arm.)

Stretch your arms out...feel the tension in the triceps muscles...and now relax, get your arms back into a comfortable position. Straighten the arms once more so that you feel the tension in the triceps muscles, straighten them out...feel that tension...and relax...Now let us concentrate on pure relaxation in the arms without any tension. Get your arms comfortable and then let them relax further and further...even when your arms seem fully relaxed, try to go that extra bit further. Try to achieve deeper and deeper levels of relaxation.

Now I want you to wrinkle up your forehead. Wrinkle it up tight, tighter and tighter...and now stop wrinkling your forehead, relax and smooth it out. Try to picture the entire forehead becoming smoother as the relaxation increases. Now frown and crease your brows and study your brow and increase the tension. Let go of the tension again...smooth out the forehead once more. Now close your eyes tighter and tighter...feel that tension...and relax your eyes. Keep your eyes closed gently and comfortably and notice the relaxation. Now clench your jaws, bite your teeth together, study the tension round the jaws...Relax your jaws now. Let your lips part slightly, appreciate the relaxation...Now press the tongue hard against the roof of your mouth. Look for the tension...Now let your tongue return to a comfortable and relaxed position. Purse your lips; press your lips together tighter and tighter...Relax the lips. Note the contrast between tension and relaxation. Feel the relaxation all over your face, all over your forehead and scalp, eyes, lips, tongue and throat...Let the relaxation progress further and further.

Now attend to your neck muscles. Press your head back as far as it can go and feel the tension in your neck. Roll it to the right now and feel the tension shift, roll it to the left...Straighten your head and bring it forward. Press your chin against your chest. Let your head return to a comfortable position and study the relaxation position. Let the relaxation spread up and down. Shrug your shoulders right up, hold that tension...hold it. Now drop your shoulders and feel the relaxation. Neck and shoulders relaxed, shrug your shoulders again and move them around. Bring your shoulders up and back. Feel the tension in your shoulders and in your upper back. Now drop your shoulders once more and relax...let the relaxation spread deep into your shoulders right into the back muscles. Relax your neck and throat and your jaws as the pure relaxation takes over and grows deeper, deeper, ever deeper...keep on relaxing like that...Feel that comfortable heaviness that accompanies relaxation. Breathe easily and freely in and out. Notice how the relaxation increases as you exhale...as you breathe out just feel that relaxation. Now breathe right in and fill your lungs. Inhale deeply and hold your breath. Study the tension...now exhale. Let the walls of your chest go loose and push the air out automatically. Continue relaxing and breathe freely and gently. Feel the relaxation and enjoy it. With the rest of your body as relaxed as possible fill your lungs again. Breathe in deeply and hold it again, hold it…that's fine. Breathe out and appreciate the relief…Now just breathe normally. Continue relaxing your chest and let the relaxation spread to your back, shoulders, neck and arms. Merely let go and enjoy the relaxation.

Now let's pay attention to your abdominal muscles, your stomach area. Tighten your stomach muscles and make your abdomen hard. Notice the tension…and relax…Let the muscles loosen and notice the contrast. Once more press and tighten your stomach muscles. Hold the tension and study it…and relax…

Notice the general well-being that comes with relaxing your stomach. Now draw your stomach in, pull the muscles right in and notice the feeling…pull them right in…now relax again. Let your stomach out. Continue breathing normally and easily and feel the gentle massaging action all over your chest and stomach. Now pull your stomach in and again hold the tension. Now push out and tense like that, hold the tension…Once more pull in and feel the tension…now relax your stomach fully. Let the tension dissolve as the relaxation grows deeper. Each time you breathe out notice the rhythmic relaxation both in your lungs and in your stomach. Notice how your chest and stomach relax more and more. Try and let go of all contractions anywhere in your body. Just let the tension leave.

Now direct your attention to your lower back. Arch up your back, make your lower back quite hollow and feel the tension along your spine…and settle down comfortably again, relaxing the lower back…Just arch your back up and feel the tension as you do so. Try and keep the rest of your body as relaxed as possible. Try and localise the tension throughout the lower back area…Relax once more, relaxing further and further…Relax your lower back, relax your upper back, spread the relaxation to your stomach, chest, shoulders, arm and facial area, these parts relaxing further and further and further and ever deeper. Let all the tension leave you.

Now finally I want you to flex your buttocks and thighs. Flex your thighs by pressing down your heels as hard as you can, press them down…now relax and note the difference. Straighten your knees and flex your thigh muscles again. Hold the tension…now relax your hips and thighs…

Allow the relaxation to proceed on its own. Press your feet and toes downwards away from your face so that your calf muscles become tense. Study that tension…now relax your feet and calves. This time bend your feet towards your face so that you feel tension in your shins…bring your toes right up. Relax again. Keep on relaxing for a while…Now let yourself relax further all over. Relax your feet, ankles, calves and shins, knees, thighs, buttocks and hips. Feel the heaviness of your lower body as you relax still further. Now spread the relaxation to your stomach, waist and lower back. Let go more and more. Feel that relaxation all over. Let it proceed to your upper back, chest, shoulders and arms and right to the tips of your fingers. Keep relaxing more and more deeply. Make sure that no tension has crept into your throat. Relax your neck and your jaws and all your facial muscles. Keep relaxing your whole body like that for a while. Let yourself relax...

Now you can become twice as relaxed as you are merely by taking a really deep breath and slowly breathing out. Take in that deep breath, hold it, now breathe out... Now take normal breaths. As you do so you will find that your body gets even more heavy, even more relaxed, and as it gets heavier so it gets warmer and warmer so you feel more and more sleepy and as you feel warm and heavy you feel even more sleepy. Your whole body feels pleasantly relaxed, all the tension has left it. Just experience that feeling, the lovely feeling of heaviness and warmth and sleepiness – a lovely relaxed sensation. Your whole body feels so heavy it seems impossible to move it. So heavy you just want to go to sleep. Your eyes are now tightly closed, very tightly closed, you feel so heavy you feel you cannot open them. There is no need to try and open them, just let that heaviness go throughout the body.

Let the tension flow out completely as you feel more and more sleepy... more and more sleepy... more and more sleepy. Just let go completely, let go altogether as you go off into a deep sleep, a deep, deep sleep. Just let yourself go to sleep, go to sleep... go to sleep... go to sleep.

Passive Muscle Relaxation

Make sure you are comfortable, sitting or lying with your eyes closed. Relax your arms by your sides and have your legs uncrossed. While I am talking to you it is important that you focus on the word '**relax**'. Let the relaxation flow over you and deepen at its own pace. Keep your breathing regular, shallow and relaxed and notice how when you breathe out you relax a little more. Breathe in and out through your nose and each time you breathe out relax further still. Keep your breathing steady, regular and relaxed and concentrate all the time on the word 'relax' each time your breathe out. Close your eyes and just let yourself relax and unwind. Concentrate on the word 'relax' and let the feeling of relaxation take over. Keep your breathing shallow and relaxed. Every time you breathe out relax a little more. Just relax as deeply as you can and let all the tensions ease away from your body. Comfortable and relaxed, heavy and content, no tension in your hands or arms. Let your hands and arms unwind completely. No tension in your shoulders, let your shoulders drop and relax. As your shoulders relax your neck feels less tense and the muscles in your neck unwind completely. There is no tension in your forehead. Smooth out your forehead, let your eyebrows droop and relax. Your eyes feel heavy and relaxed with your eyelids lightly closed. And now your jaw. Your jaw feels pleasantly relaxed, teeth slightly apart, let your jaw unwind more and more. Feel the relief of letting go...and as you feel more and more heavy and warm and relaxed your tongue becomes free of tension. Let your tongue drop down to the bottom of your mouth and relax completely...Relax your tongue and throat. Your lips and face are now feeling completely relaxed...lips lightly together, no pressure between them. Let the muscles in your face unwind and let go, no tension in your face...just let it relax more and more, more and more...heavy and relaxed...No tension in your chest. Keep your breathing shallow and relaxed and each time you breathe out concentrate on the word 'relax'. Let your body relax a little more. Your stomach muscles feel heavy and warm, let them loosen and relax.

Now think of your hips and back. As you breathe out they become pleasantly warm and heavy, free from tightness. Just let the tension flow out. Keep on breathing evenly in and out. See how you are becoming more and more relaxed...no tension in your legs...feel the tension ease away from your legs and relax them completely. Now continue this feeling throughout the whole of your body. Carry on and let your body unwind more and more deeply as you become more and more deeply relaxed...breathing relaxed and at ease. Focus on the word 'relax' and every time you breathe out relax a little more. You are sinking deeper and deeper, and becoming more and more relaxed. Just carry on letting go...enjoy the feeling of relaxation. Your whole body lets go as you become more and more relaxed, as your breathing becomes more and more easy. Your body feels heavy and relaxed, warm and free of tension. All your tension has gone, you feel pleasantly warm, relaxed and content.

11

Cognitive therapies

P. T. James

Introduction

Cognitive approaches to pain management are concerned with the way an individual thinks about his pain. These thoughts include beliefs about the cause of the pain, the threat of illness and incapacity, and the effects of treatment (*see* Chapter 3). They largely determine what help is sought and what treatments will be accepted, and they affect the mood of the sufferer. In chronic conditions such cognitions or beliefs clearly have a highly influential role in determining how an individual interacts with the medical services, and how he adjusts to his illness. However, these beliefs on cognitions are not necessarily logical or accurate. Even if they are correct it may be disadvantageous to dwell on them. The aim of the cognitive approach is to identify unhelpful beliefs that may have developed since the onset of pain and then employ techniques to change them.

The basis of cognitive therapy in chronic pain is that erroneous beliefs are identified, challenged and reassessed. A more realistic evaluation of the causes, effect, and course of the condition is made. The therapist cannot prescribe the 'best way to think', but comments on apparent illogicalities in what the patient says about his pain and behaviour, and encourages the sufferer to test out his beliefs by seeing how well they are in keeping with the prevailing evidence. Although there are some highly structured, formal methods of cognitive therapy, any person working in a Pain Clinic has the opportunity to discuss beliefs about the mechanisms of pain with patients. An approach of listening and asking open-ended questions is usually able to identify the most influential beliefs of the patient. The Pain Clinic professionals, as authority figures, have a good opportunity to change beliefs through information and education. The nurse or physiotherapist, during the time that they have structured contact with the patient, will have ample opportunity to check any maladaptive thinking through normal conversation. In these ways erroneous beliefs may be changed.

However, the health worker should avoid directly confronting the patient with such statements as 'You are making your pain worse by your attitude', or 'You are thinking negatively' without a willingness to both fully explain the process and to collaborate with the patient in bringing about change. It is all too easy for the highly trained professional to forget the limited opportunities the lay person has to learn about the anatomy and physiology of nerves and muscles. The person in pain strongly wishes to find out more about the cause of his pain so that he can fully understand it. In the absence of adequate information from experts he tends to provide his own explanation for this problem. He will consult family or friends who often make a number of unwarranted statements in good faith, which then become set beliefs.

The consequences of these systematic cognitive errors can affect the outcome considerably (*see* Chapter 3).

Why beliefs and cognitions matter

In acute medicine diagnosis and treatment can often be conducted successfully with only minimal attention to the individual's own beliefs about his condition. There is usually a recommended plan of treatment described in textbooks, which is widely shared. The exact nature of this does not have to be communicated to the patient provided sufficient compliance is established and/or the natural healing process can continue unhindered. This being said, the more a patient understands about his illness the more effective treatment techniques will be.

With a chronic condition like pain, the prevailing pain-related beliefs (pain evaluation) of the individual become crucial, as these largely determine actions and emotions and hence can give rise to inappropriate behaviour and excessive emotional distress (*see* Chapter 3). Although there may still be hope of a cure for some chronic conditions, the major goal in most patients is to minimize any disability and facilitate adjustment to a new life style with its permanent handicaps.

In Figure 11.1 the importance of the role of beliefs in determining the impact of pain on an individual is depicted. This model illustrates that the intensity and quality of noxious sensation plays only a small role. For example, a head pain attributed to muscle tension will generate an entirely different reaction from pain attributed to a brain tumour. The point to remember is that each individual has many hours to engage in 'self-dialogue', especially if daily routine and sleeping cycles are disrupted. A few seconds of worrying about the pain through a misunderstanding can directly increase distress and

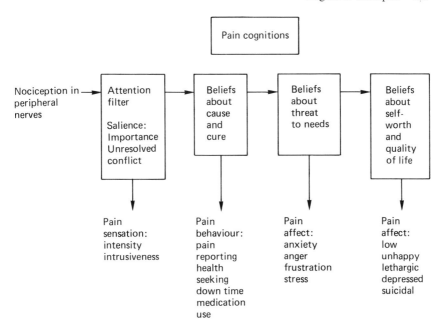

Figure 11.1 *Role of cognitions in chronic pain.*

pain behaviour. As the pain is magnified in this way the individual may believe that inactivity or bed rest is the best response for this. This may further exacerbate the pain and may even produce pathological organic changes which are difficult to reverse easily. In short, it can be seen that beliefs can have a profound effect on outcome in chronic pain.

Explaining and understanding pain

It is a difficult task to explain to a subject exactly why he is getting pain. Pain is entirely subjective and so cannot directly be assessed or categorized. Many patients find it difficult to articulate the nature of their pain, are aware of their problem in conveying this, and believe that they have not therefore been understood adequately. They consequently believe that the expert's explanations about the cause of their pain is not accurate as it is based on incomplete information. Communication can be improved by the use of pain drawings or visual analogue scales, and by noting what the patient says about factors that increase or decrease pain. The clinician can check how well the patient feels he has been understood by asking: 'How well do you think we have understood the nature of your pain?' 'Are there aspects of your pain which do not fit with our explanation?'

Patients have their own models in their head about what is causing their pain, i.e. their own 'illness representation'. Even if the clinicians cannot explain fully the pain, they are usually able enough to alter the patient's illness representation if this is based on misconceptions. However, for various reasons, including poor communication skills or inadequate alternative models, the patient may retain his own erroneous view. This is made less likely if the clinicians have understood the patient's own illness representation and demonstrated that understanding, and as far as possible acknowledged the patient's own views when providing a 'professional' explanation. Suggested lead questions by the therapist include: 'What ideas do you have about the cause of your pain?' 'What do your family or friends think is causing your pain?' 'So a number of possibilities have gone through your mind about the cause. Have I got them right, they include...' 'Your theory about the pain is in part right because...'.

We learn a lot vicariously from the experiences of others, either through the media or in real life. We identify with people, or see similarities. This gives us ideas about action to take, even though in the company of directive and authoritative clinicians we may be reluctant to divulge them. To encourage both appropriate health-seeking behaviour and compliance it is as well to disabuse people of their unhelpful ideas and capitalize on their sensible ones. So the clinician may ask 'What ideas do you have about what can be done to help you?' 'Have you heard of, or know, anyone with a similar problem? What help did they get?'

Patients are bound to have difficulties understanding their condition if after extensive diagnostic tests the clinicians have not themselves reached a conclusion. In such circumstances clinicians may offer their best explanation without sufficiently stressing the tentative nature of their model, often because they wish to reduce the anxiety associated with uncertainty. Unfortunately this can lead to contradictory models being offered by different clinicians. As a result the patient does not know whom or what to believe. Pain Clinics can help by acknowledging to patients that this occurs, and by being prepared to tolerate the ambiguity. The following examples illustrate the messages which in the short term may not be the most reassuring, but in the long term are likely to be the most helpful. 'We cannot be sure what is happening but the most probable explanation is...' 'How does that fit the facts you have?' 'At this stage we can only guess at what is happening. Two main possibilities exist... You're probably disappointed we cannot be more exact'.

One critical misunderstanding is concerned with the capacity of treatments to 'cure' chronic pain. From the patient's perspective the loss of hope and pessimism about the future that comes from switching from an 'acute' to a 'chronic' illness representation has a major impact. Apart from the emotional distress associated with the realization that a permanent disability is present, in many aspects similar to a bereavement reaction, the sufferer also recognizes sooner or later that he will have to manage his problems to at least some extent on his own without relying on professional help. Appropriate help at this time of transition can encourage adaptive styles of coping, and help people set their new expectations to realistic levels. The size of this task needs to be assessed to see how much help the patient will need. 'What are you realistically hoping for in the future in terms of your pain?' 'Taking a pessimistic view, if your pain were not to improve over the next five years what would happen to you?'

Finally in this section we can learn to identify the ways in which people misunderstand by considering five typical errors we all make in our thinking. These can be appropriately applied to pain.

Error	Example
Selective abstraction	Noticing only when the pain is bad and not remembering the good times
Overgeneralization	Difficulty during one task on one day gets exaggerated into it being a problem always, and on other tasks too
Dichotomous reasoning	Either I'm well or I'm very ill, the pain will be cured or get worse
Personalization	It's my fault that the pain is not improving, and that I cannot do more to help
Arbitrary inference	Jumping to the conclusion, on insufficient evidence, that the condition will rapidly deteriorate

Negative thinking

It is easy to comprehend how misunderstanding by the patient leads to erroneous beliefs. What is often of more importance in determining maintenance of pain and pain behaviour are negative thoughts. Dwelling on adverse experiences or exaggerating the adverse experiences resulting from the pain are typical negative thoughts that can affect the course of chronic pain. Although ideally we should replace this form of disadvantageous thinking with more positive thoughts it may not always be possible to do this immediately, and so the therapist should encourage activities which by occupying attention necessarily displace negative thinking.

Typical negative thoughts include perceived threats to well-being, relationships, role, control of emotions and self-esteem because of pain. They involve beliefs about poor body image, self-esteem, that life has little pleasure to offer, and that the future is bleak. The major problem is that negative thinking leads to more negative thinking, a downward spiral which needs to be arrested. If people have too much time to think negatively they can become clinically depressed and suicidal.

Examples of typical negative thinking include:

1 'My condition is getting worse so they can't have found the real cause yet'.

2 'My pain is killing me; it must be more than a trapped nerve'.

3 'This pain is like my aunt's, and she died of cancer'.

4 'This pulling pain feels as though something is tearing. I'll have to go to bed for a week to let it heal'.

5 'I can't cope with the pain, it will drive me crazy'.

6 'I am still convinced I should have another X-ray'.

7 'I read about an ultrasound scan, couldn't that be tried?'

8 'My GP keeps telling me there is nothing else to do, so have I just got to suffer?'

9 'I will try anything as long as it takes my pain away'.

10 'No one wants to know me now, I'm useless'.

11 'There is nothing I can do well.'

Certain styles of negative thinking may be discerned which need to be checked (e.g. Catalano, 1987). Engaging in these ways of thinking are generally unhelpful and so should be avoided.

Blaming	– others for cause or worsening of pain without taking responsibility
Shoulds	– not might or could do things but should do them leads to unrealistic expectations
Unrealistic control	– seeing others in control of your life, e.g. doctors
Led by emotions	– because you feel something it must be true
Dark glasses	– noticing only problems and the pain, filtering out the bright things
Expecting justice	– believing it is not fair to suffer chronic pain

Changing beliefs by listening

When people are given an opportunity to talk through their thoughts, especially when the listener is non-judgmental and facilitative, then they can make progress in developing and changing their ideas. This is especially the case when the attendent emotions are ventilated too. The listener can paraphrase tentatively what the patient is saying, so allowing the patient to check out how realistic or useful is his way of thinking. Consider the following example:

Patient   – It hurts me too much to go fishing, so even though I used to really enjoy it, I'll never go again.

Therapist – So you think that you'll never go fishing again because the pain stops you from enjoying it, is that right?

Patient   – Well I wouldn't be able to fish for hours on end, I'd have to do it in stages.

Thought stopping

The aim of thought stopping is to disrupt certain negative thinking as soon as possible, and replace the unwanted thoughts with those that are more constructive. Once the rationale has been explained the patient is taught to recognize 'outlawed' thoughts, and then displace them. The following suggestions can be helpful in this context:

1 take a slow breath out.

2 imagine a blackboard being cleared.

3 say something positive – I can manage my pain
                                        – I have control
                                        – I am okay

4 add a cheering or motivating statement; the language can be as strong as the person wants
                                        – stop this negative rubbish
                                        – to hell with this stuff
                                        – get lost you moaning minnies

5 engage in some new and neutral activity, a list of which could be prepared in advance – something to listen to or read
                                        – a plan to make
                                        – a memory to return to
                                        – a problem to solve
                                        – a story/poem to sing/recite aloud

Cognitive therapy

More formal cognitive therapy requires individuals to identify situations or *Activating* (A) events which then causes them to engage in certain self-statements or *Beliefs* (B). The *Consequence* (C) of these beliefs on mood is then noted. Finally, this leads to *Dispute* (D) of these situationally activated events to change the outcome. As part of therapy the individual keeps a diary of events and beliefs, and the therapist then collaborates with him to challenge the prevailing negative beliefs. The patient is therefore learning to break down their experiences into A's, B's and C's, and then applying D's to change the sequence.

An example of an ABCD construction is given. Mr. X, a man with chronic mechanical back pain, is unable to do the decorating and watches his wife complete the task. This *Activating* event leads to *Beliefs* such as, 'I should do that', 'I am useless', 'Things are never going to improve', and 'I'll end up with everything having to be done for me'. The *Consequences* of this obviously worsen mood and generate more negative thinking and memories. To *Disrupt* these Mr. X challenges the evidence for each belief, e.g. 'Other wives enjoy decorating, and mine seems to as well', 'I can still do most things', 'There is no evidence that things will get worse', and 'Look at other people who develop a new life despite their pain'.

Cognitive coping strategies

Increasing tolerance to pain

The patient is encouraged to work for pain tolerance, not pain avoidance. He needs to recognize that pain is going to be a factor that will influence his life, but it need not be the most important one. It is not a sign of further physical damage if it persists in its present form; it is only if there is a dramatic change in its quality or intensity that further professional attention should be sought. It should be seen as unfortunate but unavoidable.

The sufferer's task is to minimize the disability and to apply a range of coping strategies whilst living his life as normally as possible. These are likely to include relaxation and cognitive distraction.

Active role and reconceptualization

The aim is for the 'patient' to progress to 'non-patient' status by assuming more responsibility for the management of his condition. During this process he is bound to gain a sense of increased control.

This change has been described as 'reconceptualization', an important underlying aim to all psychological therapeutic endeavours. Reconceptualization involves a change in beliefs about where the power to alter pain sensation and behaviour rests, an integral part of which includes an alteration in the individual's perception that he can indeed influence and change his circumstances in some way.

It is a radical approach which involves the individual solving his own problems rather than simply being the passive recipient of advice. The patient's beliefs in the power of medical treatment may make this difficult, especially if investigations are still under way.

All health workers working with chronic pain patients can aid this process. When helping the individual to 'reconceptualize', the therapist is at all times trying to encourage new ideas from the sufferer about the factors underlying his pain. It is important not to be prescriptive in recommending any new therapy. The professional should apply these in such a way that this process can be encouraged, e.g. 'Here is an approach you might like to try' rather than 'Do this five times each week and let us know what happens'.

Mood management

In the normal course of events people have the luxury of being able to experience fluctuating levels of stress, anxiety or unhappiness without any long-term adverse effects. In chronic pain strong emotions often need to be avoided because of their direct effect in increasing pain sensation. However, pain in itself is a natural stressor, and can lead to demoralization and unhappiness. So patients are already in a more emotionally labile state. If this emotional vulnerability can be lessened then pain sensation and pain affect will both be reduced. Although relaxation is helpful in managing some aspects of anxiety and stress, the most direct way is to control the direction of internal thoughts. There are, in addition, more general stress management techniques involving physical fitness, pacing, diet, sleep routines and avoidance of procrastination, as well as initiating appropriate support from others. One or more of these can all be adopted.

Positive thinking

Unfortunately there are situations where a patient's beliefs are pessimistic yet are quite realistic. The unhelpful emotions or behaviour that are engendered are to be expected under these circumstances. In these cases where there are grounds for believing that the prognosis is going to become worse with increasing disability, the patient requires to develop a new set of more adaptive beliefs in order to improve his mood. It is worth noting that the majority of people normally want to be given information about their condition even if the news is not good because knowledge is better than uncertainty.

In these circumstances it is surprisingly often found that patients develop unrealistically optimistic beliefs about their future. However, because they are positive in their attitudes a good outcome in terms of emotional adjustment usually ensues and disability is minimized. This style of coping should not be actively encouraged by the health care worker in an overt way as it is important that false information is not given out by the professional. However, in view of its beneficial effects it is a technique of coping that the therapist would not wish to undermine. Although there is some evidence that the durability of such attitudes are a little tenuous, if it appears to be working for the patient it would be cruel and unnecessary to disavow the patient's beliefs.

Positive Imagery

Imagery is one of a number of creative ways of diverting attention away from pain or changing its nature. Its use is of particular value in subjects who are able to imagine previously experienced feelings and situations easily. During deep relaxation this ability can be tested. The techniques have been described by Turk, Meichenbaum and Genest (1983) and used by many clinicians. Patients often need considerable help at first in using imagery successfully, and may need information of how other patients have coped with this sort of technique.

Imagery can be used in a number of ways:

1   Imaginative inattention

The subject is asked under relaxation to imagine a scene in which pain is absent, e.g. walking effortlessly in the countryside, lying in the sun.

2   Transformation of pain

During deep relaxation or hypnosis the subject is asked to imagine pain sensation as something else such as numbness, or to minimize these sensations as trivial or irrelevant.

3   Transformation of context

It is suggested to the subject that the cause of his present symptoms be altered to anything new, e.g. sports injury, war scene, situation where others must not know of the pain, etc.

Attentional diversion

The aim is to occupy the attention away from pain, but without having to rely on artificial distractors. Apart from the imagery techniques discussed, and the many relaxation approaches discussed in Chapter 10, the following can also be developed as a skill. Concentration is required. The following are suggested:

1 Focusing on the immediate environment, noticing details that would normally be ignored (e.g. colours, shapes, sizes, texture, noises, smells, contrasts, similarities).

2 Concentrating on mental activities, plans, problems, sums and memories.

3 Paying attention to alternative bodily sensations such as warmth, sensations when breathing and feelings of touch.

It is also useful to have a wide range of sources of stimulation available to use as distractors, e.g. interesting magazines, short stories, music.

Conclusion

Cognitive approaches are helpful in most patients who attend pain clinics. Most patients hold a number of false beliefs about their pain and if these remain unaltered after information and discussion, more structured cognitive therapy should be considered. If maladaptive thoughts cannot be changed, then they can be actively displaced by more neutral or distracting thoughts. Clearly the patient has to be given responsibility for doing this. However, all workers in the Pain Clinic should be able to detect disparaging and pessimistic statements by patients about themselves and their future and challenge these by using some of the coping strategies described in this chapter.

Bibliography

Catalano, E. M. (1987) *The Chronic Pain Control Workbook*. New Harbinger Publications Inc., Oakland, Calif.

Hanson, R. W. and Gerber, K. E. (1990) *Coping with Chronic Pain*. Guilford Press, New York

Holzman, A. D. and Turk, D. C. (1986) *Pain Management: A Handbook of Psychological Treatment Approaches*. Pergamon Press, New York

Philips, H. C. (1988) *The Psychological Management of Chronic Pain – A Manual*. Springer, New York

Turk, D. C., Meichenbaum, D.H. and Genest, M. (1983) *Pain and Behavioural Medicine: A Cognitive Behavioural Perspective*. Guilford Press, New York

12

Hypnosis
S. P. Tyrer

Hypnosis is an altered state of awareness or consciousness in which the subject becomes more receptive to suggestions. These suggestions can be made by another person or by the subject himself. Hypnosis is not new, such techniques have been used for at least 4000 years. In ancient Egypt soothsayers induced a trance-like state in patients with painful and other symptoms. The dramatic effects that sometimes occurred persuaded many that religious influences were at work and there are references in the Talmud and the Bible to 'the laying-on of hands'. This is the origin of faith-healing.

Although these early writings showed that hypnosis could be used to relieve pain and other symptoms, the medical profession were for many years very dubious of its efficacy. This was due in no small part to the influence of an Austrian faith-healer called Franz Mesmer who believed that his hypnotic powers were due to an invisible force called 'animal magnetism', which was influenced by the configuration of the stars and planets. Mesmer's influence was widespread (the word 'mesmerism' actually derives from his name), and when his interpretation of the cause of hypnotic suggestibility was doubted by scientists, the reputation of hypnosis was undermined. Thus, in the mid-19th century when Ward, a Nottingham surgeon, amputated a thigh under hypnosis, without any sign of distress on the part of the patient, the account of the operation was suppressed by other surgeons. It was not until 1955 that the British Medical Association gave approval for hypnosis to be taught in medical schools; the American Medical Association followed 3 years later. There are now regular courses run by the British Society of Medical and Dental Hypnosis for doctors and dentists.

The nature of the hypnotic state

Braid, a Scottish physician, first used the word hypnosis in 1844; it derives from the Greek word for sleep, *hypnos*. However, later he realized that subjects in a hypnotic trance were not asleep but were very relaxed and highly suggestible.

Between 60 and 70% of adults are hypnotizable to some degree. One in seven are highly suggestible and it is from this section of the population that those subjects who perform extraordinary acts under the glare of media exposure are found. A hypnotized subject, although relaxed, is actually focusing closely on everything that the therapist is saying. It is as though all other stimuli have been reduced or cut off so that attention is concentrated on one thing only.

It is not easy to predict which subjects are hypnotizable. Although the subject must be willing to try the technique and to have confidence in the person employing it the degree of hypnosis obtained cannot be predicted from these factors. The experience of the person using hypnosis is a factor in determining hypnotizability although this may be partly reflected in the faith of the patient in the therapist concerned. Only patients who are able to focus and concentrate will be good subjects and, despite lay impressions to the contrary, the mean intelligence of subjects found to be easily hypnotizable is above average. Although Charcot, a French neurologist, stated at the end of the 19th century that only hysterical patients could be rendered hypnotizable, this has now been shown to be clearly false and easily hypnotizable subjects neither have more hysterical personalities nor are more prone to hysterical mechanisms than others. This being said, patients who develop conversion symptoms are by definition more suggestible and may under hypnosis lose their handicaps. Good subjects are highly suggestible and suggestibility is a factor in predisposing to the mechanism of dissociation, the mechanism involved in hysterical reactions.

Hypnosis in pain

Hypnosis may be used in any painful condition or procedure, whether this be acute or chronic. It may be the only form of pain relief but it is more commonly given in addition to other techniques of pain relief. There is a widespread misconception by many people that subjects that respond to hypnosis must have 'pain in the mind', or that the fact that hypnosis works means that their pain does not truly have a physical basis. This is not so; the most important factor in determining reduction of pain by hypnosis is the degree of hypnotizability of the subject. Although there is some suggestion that acute pains are more effectively treated than chronic pains the origin of the pain is not a factor which usually affects the level of response to hypnosis. Effective muscular relaxation is one of the most important ingredients in success in hypnosis in pain, but distraction and the capacity to concentrate on non-painful topics are also important.

Hypnosis has been used successfully in chronic pain due to cancer, burns, headaches, chronic dental pain and phantom limb pains in particular, although hypnosis can be used for any painful condition. Children are much more readily hypnotizable than adults and this method of analgesia is often preferred for acute procedures, e.g. the insertion of needles. In adults, phantom limb pains, which are often difficult to control by other means, show a gratifying reduction with hypnosis.

Factors determining response in hypnosis

In a subject that is readily hypnotizable, the induction of hypnosis is surprisingly easy. What is needed for success is belief in the therapist by the subject, expectations that the treatment will be beneficial and skill on the part of the therapist. The technique of hypnosis can be learned by instruction and observation of experienced hypnotists. However, any person wishing to use hypnosis widely, particularly with patients, is recommended to attend a course organized by an appropriate professional body. In Great Britain, the British Society of Medical and Dental Hypnosis is such an organization whilst in the USA the Council on Mental Health of the American Medical Association carries out similar functions. A short list of organizations that run training courses in the UK and USA is given at the end of this chapter.

A commonly held belief is that in hypnosis it is necessary for the subject to be unaware of what the therapist is doing otherwise the patient is not hypnotized. Although the hallmark of stage hypnosis is to render their subjects unaware of their actions under hypnosis this is not normally valuable when hypnosis is used as a therapeutic modality, particularly in chronic pain. For instance, it may well be possible for the hypnotist to completely remove a pain during the hypnotic session. Unfortunately, it is usual for pain to recur within a short time after a successful treatment in the therapist's office. There are a number of reasons why this is so.

Hypnosis by a therapist is performed on a patient in a passive role. The patient believes that only the therapist is able to treat the pain successfully and their expectation is that outside the hypnosis session their pain will remain. Pain is relieved by hypnosis because of relaxation and distraction and it may simply be that the patient is too tense and/or preoccupied with his pain for reduction in pain intensity following the session to be maintained. It is possible that the pain experienced is as a result of, or is being maintained by, emotional conflicts or is being rewarded in a direct or subtle way. In these cases it may be necessary to delve further into the factors that precipitated the pain.

It is possible for some degree of pain relief following the session to be obtained if the hypnotist uses a technique called post-hypnotic suggestion during the time the patient is hypnotized. The therapist suggests to the subject that the pains will not recur when the hypnotic trance is removed. This may have some effect for a time but post-hypnotic suggestions of this nature do not often last longer than a few days at most. It is possible for the subject to continue to see the hypnotist at weekly or fortnightly intervals so as to facilitate further post-hypnotic suggestion but this is an extensive and time-consuming procedure.

Of greater value is self-hypnosis. If the subject remains in touch with the therapist during the hypnotic trance, the feelings experienced by the subject can be remembered and produced by the use of self-hypnosis or autohypnosis. This is not complicated. It simply involves the patient directly relaxing himself using the same technique that he has learnt from the therapist. For it to be successful, it is essential that the subject be aware of the feelings he has during hypnotic induction so that he can appreciate the feelings and sensations that result when he is in an hypnotic trance.

Induction of hypnosis

The first task of the hypnotist is to determine the degree of hypnotizability of the patient with chronic pain. He therefore aims to induce an hypnotic trance and determine the degree of hypnotizability during the session. This is usually the sole purpose of the initial interview and it is not necessary to reduce the level of pain experienced by the patient at this session. All induction procedures involve the subject fixing their attention on a particular object. A visual object is usually chosen, but senses in other modalities could theoretically be used. The commonest procedure, and one which is easily employable in the physician's office, is to fix on some particular point in the room at eye level height. A small coloured disk on the wall may be all that is required. In the Newcastle Pain Relief Clinic, a swinging pendulum is used, the speed and amplitude of the oscillation being gradually reduced during the procedure.

The subject is asked to sit in a relaxed position facing the visual stimulus concerned and asked to gaze fixedly at this spot. The hypnotist then gradually relaxes the person by asking him to breathe increasingly more deeply and informing him that he is becoming progressively more relaxed. As the subject does so, it becomes increasingly difficult for him to focus on the object concerned, his eyelids become tired and the hypnotist suggests that he may be falling asleep. The subject may then find that he is unable to keep his eyes open and further deeper relaxation is carried out at this time.

A number of techniques can then be used to determine how well the subject is likely to respond to which forms of suggestion. In practice, the ability of the subject to:

1 Imagine alternative feelings or experiences and,

2 Produce a motor response to direct suggestion.

are of most importance. There are a large number of ways in which these procedures can be carried out. What follows is a description of the procedures used by the author and others in Newcastle.

The capacity for the subject to experience imagery is usually determined in the following manner. The extent of visual imagery is measured by the therapist suggesting that there will be a walk down a short staircase which will intensify the relaxed feelings. The staircase is described and then the subject is asked to walk down the stairs, counting them as they do so. The vividness of the experience of the subject when questioned after the session helps to determine the extent of visual imagery. The subject's feet may move during the session as though they are descending the staircase. In the same way, the intensity of the feelings experienced by the subject when a suggestion is made of lying on a beach in warm sunlight may be used therapeutically if pain is relieved by heat. Alternatively, tactile imagery may be used.

Production of a motor response should also be attempted at the first session. The effects of suggesting that the subject's arm is gradually becoming lighter, as though it is being raised upwards by invisible balloons, helps to ascertain the degree of motor response to direct suggestibility. If patients respond well to this form of suggestion, it may be appropriate to suggest that they reduce their pain by turning down a gauge depicting their level of pain, or to move the pain experienced from one part of the body to another. In some instances, where patients have been dependent on physical aids, it may be possible for them to behave as though they were using such an aid, whereas in fact they are not.

In this way, the first session both determines whether or not the subject is likely to respond to further hypnotic sessions and how these should be best conducted in order to have the maximum effect. In all, some five to eight sessions are usually given, although the number is dependent upon the problem concerned and the benefit obtained. It is valuable after the third or fourth session to encourage the use of self-hypnosis. In order to assess this, a relaxation tape by the therapist may be given to the patient after the second or third session in order to aid their own self-hypnosis. Some therapists record a session with the subject; extraneous noises often render such recordings of inadequate quality and a pre-existing tape, although not specifically designed for the subject concerned, is often of more benefit.

Conclusion

Hypnosis is not suitable for everybody but can bring benefits both in organic and psychogenic pain. The reasons for using it can range from simply aiding relaxation to finding out more about the origin and persistence of painful memories. It has the advantage of not causing any deleterious side-effects if carried out by an experienced therapist. It should in virtually all cases be accompanied by self-hypnotic instruction so that further treatments can be carried out by the patient himself.

Organizations providing training in hypnotism

In the UK

British Society of Medical and Dental Hypnotists
42 Links Road
Ashted
Surrey

British Society of Hypnotherapists
51 Queen Anne Street
London W1M 9FA

Therapy Training College
8/10 Balaclava Road
Birmingham B14 7S6

In the USA

American Society of Clinical Hypnosis
2400E. Devon Avenue
Suite 218 Des Plaines
Illinois 60018

Society for Clinical and Experimental Hypnosis
129A. Kings Park Drive
Liverpool
New York 13088

American Psychological Association
Division 30 – Psychological Hypnosis
1200 Seventeenth Street, N.W.
Washington DC 20036

A directory of Affiliated Societies to the International Society of Hypnosis is available from:

International Society of Hypnosis
C/O Unit for Experimental Psychiatry
111 North Fortyninth Street
Philadelphia, Pennsylvania 19139, USA

Bibliography

Hilgard, E. and Hilgard, J. (1975) *Hypnosis in the Relief of Pain.* William Kaufmann Inc., California

13

Information about pain

S. P. Tyrer

Introduction

Patients with chronic pain are often bewildered by their state and are unable to explain it. They have been seen by a multitude of doctors, have often received conflicting advice and are unsure exactly what is causing their pain and how their symptoms should be adequately managed. As with all medical problems, it is important to inform and educate the patient as far as possible about the cause of his illness and the choice of treatment. Many patients find it difficult to ask their doctors direct questions and they are often anxious and distressed at the time of their consultation and so cannot always collect their thoughts and articulate their problems clearly. As a result, erroneous impressions and faulty knowledge leads to persistence with attitudes that may further exacerbate pain.

To take an example, a 60-year-old lady I saw recently in the Pain Clinic was convinced that her pain was due to osteoporosis, an illness characterized by reduced bone density. She knew sufficient about this illness to know that there is an increased danger of fractures in this condition. As a result, she spent a good deal of her time in bed in order to reduce the possibility of falling and fracturing her limbs. In fact, prolonged bed rest increases demineralization of the bones, leading to osteoporosis. This lady had selected a mode of living which was actually making her condition worse because of her erroneous beliefs.

The need for information and education of people with chronic pain is evident. It is an essential element of all cognitive treatments in pain (*see* Chapter 11). How can this information be disseminated?

In an ideal world, the doctor concerned with the patient with chronic pain would explain the factors that have contributed to the patient's painful state and would answer all questions posed by the patient as accurately as possible. However, doctors are busy, they only have a certain amount of time in which to examine and treat the patient and under these circumstances it is all too common for the origin of the patients' problems and the use of treatments for these not to be discussed in detail. When the diagnosis is uncertain, which is frequently the case, explanation is even less likely to be forthcoming.

The doctor can overcome this problem by giving out leaflets explaining the basic features of certain conditions he treats and what treatments are available. Audio tapes have also been used in this context and are of greater benefit than reading books alone.

Patients and many otherwise well-informed doctors know very little about what activities take place in the average pain clinic. A large number of widely differing procedures are used in many pain clinics and as many of these involve technical skills the greatest educational benefit can be derived from video cassettes illustrating the work that goes on at the clinic. It is helpful for the patient to watch a video cassette of this nature while waiting for their appointment in the pain clinic. Copies to take home may also be available.

These methods, although of value, need to be supplemented with subsequent discussion with the doctor about specific problems presented by the patient. On the whole, patients expect and like simple explanations and consequently ask questions such as: 'Is my pain due to a slipped disc or not?', 'If my X-ray shows spondylitis does that not mean that this is the cause of my neck pain?'. In practice, a large number of factors contribute to the extent of chronic pain and it is rarely possible to give 'black and white' answers. In the same way, the doctor cannot make absolute judgements about the likely effectiveness of the treatments or manoeuvres in the treatment of chronic pain. He can only give an idea of the likelihood of certain treatments improving the patient's pain.

For this reason, amongst others, it is valuable for the patient to write down a list of questions that he wishes to ask the doctor. These should be phrased as far as possible in such a manner that the doctor is able to answer them effectively. Questions such as 'How likely is this treatment to improve my backache?' and 'Do the side-effects of this treatment sometimes/often outweigh its benefits?' are more likely to be answered accurately than questions such as 'Will it make me better?' It is often valuable for the patient to bring a close relative with him to the clinic when he is seen by the doctor. The doctor usually wishes to talk to a close associate of the patient and the patient may wish to discuss the explanations given by the doctor with somebody they know well. Further questions may arise following discussion about these issues.

Pain education groups

As it is often difficult for doctors to explain in detail about painful conditions, some centres have developed information or education

Table 13.1 Programme for pain education class

Week 1	Introduction to Pain Clinic Origin of pain Relationship between acute and chronic pain Assessment procedures
Week 2	Surgery for pain
Week 3	Drugs used in the treatment of pain
Week 4	Anaesthetic measures
Week 5	Psychiatry and Pain
Week 6	Transcutaneous electrical nerve stimulation Acupuncture
Week 7	Physiotherapy
Week 8	Psychological treatments
Week 9	Social work intervention and disability benefits

Each of these classes is directed by a specialist in the subject concerned

groups to talk about these problems. A typical group consists of specialists from disciplines concerned with the problem from which the patients are suffering. For instance, a Back Pain Education Group might involve an orthopaedic surgeon, physiotherapist and anaesthetist.

At the Newcastle Pain Relief Clinic, which is concerned with a large variety of different painful conditions, seven specialists working in the Pain Clinic give short talks about their work to patients who wish to be informed about the origin and treatment of painful states. The speakers involved include a surgeon, physiotherapist, anaesthetist, pharmacologist, psychologist, psychiatrist and social worker. Each talks for 20 minutes or so on their topic and then there is general discussion regarding the issues raised. A leaflet concerned with the topic under discussion is distributed at the meeting. A typical programme is illustrated in Table 13.1. It is valuable for those attending these groups to come to all the meetings so that they have a comprehensive overview of the services offered by the Pain Clinic and have a clear understanding of all the factors that contribute to pain.

The composition of these groups and how they operate is a matter for local consideration. However, these groups are normally set up in such a way that they are not intended to be supportive for long periods. There is a case for groups of this sort, but their function is not concerned with information and education.

How far should patients be asked to take part in these groups or should they choose to join them if they wish? The experience of the Newcastle Pain Relief Clinic is that these groups should be part of the programme of instruction for selected patients who begin attendance at the Clinic. The groups are valuable for anybody suffering from chronic pain, but are of particular help to patients who have erroneous ideas about the pathology that is causing their own pain and who are convinced they have a serious disease despite little pathological evidence to support this. We have found that many different types of patient benefit from these groups and they may be of benefit to patients with a wide variety of painful complaints. It is not normally vital to select patients carefully for attendance at these groups. There are some individuals who, because of their personality, or because of their experiences in the hands of pain professionals, should be included in a group with other forceful personalities who are able to provide a counterweight to others' opinions. If a group becomes engrossed in attempting to solve the problems of one particular patient, the professional taking the group should redirect the discussion to more general themes.

Where to go for help

A number of organizations exist which help guide the sufferer with chronic pain and who can be contacted regarding the legal, statutory and discretionary rights of disabled people. These are listed below:

Arthritis and Rheumatism Council,
41 Eagle Street, London, WC1R 4AR.
Tel. 071 405 8572.

Association of Disabled Professionals,
The Stables, 73 Pound Road, Banstead, Surrey, SM7 2HU.
Tel. 073 73 52366.

Back Pain Association,
Grundy House, 31–33 Park Road, Teddington, Middlesex,
TW11 0AB.
Tel. 081 977 5474.

British Limbless Ex-Servicemen's Association,
Frankland Moore House, 185/7 High Road, Chadwell Heath, Essex,
RM6 6NA.
Tel. 081 590 1124/5.

British Migraine Association,
178a High Road, Byfleet, Weybridge, Surrey, KT14 7ED.
Tel. 093 23 52468.

Centre on Environment for the Handicapped,
126 Albert Street, London, NW1 7NF.
Tel. 071 267 6111, ext. 264/5.

Chest, Heart and Stroke Association,
Tavistock House North, Tavistock Square, London, WC1H 9JE.
Tel. 071 387 3012.

Consumers' Association,
14 Buckingham Street, London, WC2N 6DS.
Tel. 071 839 1222.

Disability Alliance,
1 Cambridge Terrace, London, NW1 4JL.
Tel. 071 935 4992.

Disabled Income Group,
Attlee House,
28 Commercial Road, London, E1 6LR.
Tel. 071 247 2128/6877.

Disabled Living Foundation,
380/384 Harrow Road, London, W9 2HU.
Tel. 071 289 6111.

Greater London Association for the Disabled (GLAD),
1 Thorpe Close, London, W10 5XL.
Tel. 081 960 5799.

Greater London Association for Initiatives in Disablement (GLAID),
Flat 4, 188 Ramsden Road, Balham, London, SW12.
Tel. 081 673 4310.

Joint Committee on Mobility for the Disabled,
c/o ASBAH, Tavistock House North, Tavistock Square, London,
WC1H 9JE.
Tel. 071 388 1382.

Mobility Information Service,
Copthorne Community Hall, Shelton Road, Copthorne, Shrewsbury,
SY3 8TD.
Tel. 0743 68383.

Multiple Sclerosis Society of Great Britain and Northern Ireland,
25 Effie Road, Fulham, London, SW6 1EE.
Tel. 071 381 4022/5.

Patients' Association,
Room 33, 18 Charing Cross Road, London, WC2H 0HR.
Tel. 071 240 0671.

PHAB (Physically Handicapped and Able Bodied),
42 Devonshire Street, London, W1N 1LN.
Tel. 071 637 7475.

Spinal Injuries Association,
Yeoman House, 76 St. James Lane, Muswell Hill, London, N10.
Tel. 081 444 2121.

14

Other treatment strategies (TENS and acupuncture)

J. W. Thompson

There are several forms of local treatment for the relief of pain that (i) do not involve taking drugs, (ii) are not primarily psychological, and (iii) are used by a number of different therapists. The two principal therapies concerned are acupuncture and transcutaneous electrical nerve stimulation (TENS).

Acupuncture

Acupuncture now plays an ever-increasing role in Western medicine. Willem Ten Rhijne (1647–1700), a Dutch physician who visited Nagasaki in Japan in the early 17th century, invented the European term acupuncture (*acus* = needle, *punctura* = puncture) and wrote a dissertation on the subject in 1683. However, the first recorded use of it in the West appears to have been in 1810 when Dr Berlioz, physician and father of the musical composer Hector Berlioz, applied it to the treatment of abdominal pain. Thereafter the use of acupuncture in the Western hemisphere developed independently in various countries. In France during the first half of the 19th century Volleix discovered and utilized many acupuncture points oblivious of the existence of the Chinese practice, whilst Sarlandiere developed and used an early form of electroacupuncture. In England at about the same time the physician John Churchill did much to stimulate interest in acupuncture, whilst in North America it was also being actively used. Since the latter part of the 19th century the use of acupuncture has increased steadily in the West, albeit to varying degrees in different countries. Furthermore, during the past 15–20 years there has been an enormous upsurge of interest in acupuncture which has been due to a number of developments taking place during this period. The improvement in communication between East and

West, particularly following the Cultural Revolution in China, increased the awareness of those in the West to the practice of acupuncture. This situation was given an extra boost when President Nixon visited China in 1971 and was able to see for himself (together with his physicians who accompanied him) the practice and results of acupuncture. In the same decade, the discovery in 1975 by Professor Hans Kosterlitz and Dr John Hughes of the opioid peptides produced a further surge of interest when it was realized that acupuncture might work at least in part through the release of these endogenous compounds.

Traditional Background

Acupuncture is part of traditional Chinese medicine that has probably been in existence for over 5000 years. Essentially, it involves inserting fine needles into the skin at certain specific sites called acupuncture points (acupoints). Sets of these points, each relating to a particular organ, for example, lung, liver or heart, are joined by lines to form meridians of which twelve are situated bilaterally and two are in the mid-line. According to traditional theory, the important principle is that of a dynamic balance between two opposing forces called Yin and Yang which are responsible for the flow of life energy or Chi through the meridians. When these forces are in balance the result is good health, whereas imbalance results in disease. Yin is passive and peaceful, whereas Yang is dominant and active. Examples of disorders due to an excess of Yin are depression and obesity; disorders due to an excess of Yang are anxiety and hypertension. Yin disorders are treated by using acupuncture to stimulate Yang and so restore the balance of forces; and vice versa.

Relationship between traditional Chinese acupuncture and the concepts of western medicine

To date, no convincing evidence has been forthcoming to support the existence of meridians, the life force (Chi) which flows through them either in a state of balance (health) or of imbalance (disease); or of the existence of Yin and Yang. These appear to be metaphysical concepts that have evolved out of Chinese philosophy and traditional medicine. One may ask therefore whether there is any correspondence between acupuncture points or meridians and the concepts of Western medicine? There are indeed a number of ways in which the Eastern and Western systems are related. It seems likely that in many instances acupuncture points represent sites where various nerves become more accessible to stimulation by a needle inserted through the overlying skin. Thus, a particular acupuncture 'point' may simply represent a site where a particular nerve takes a course which brings it closer to the subcutaneous tissues or to the site at which a motor nerve enters a voluntary muscle ('motor point').

Furthermore in terms of modern Western physiology, Yin can be equated approximately with the activity of the parasympathetic nervous system, and Yang with that of the sympathetic nervous system. What is certainly clear is that in spite of the untenable theories upon which acupuncture is based, Western medicine is belatedly recognizing that it can make a valuable contribution to certain areas of it.

Role of acupuncture in the treatment of chronic pain

At the outset it is important to make it clear that acupuncture is no more a panacea for the treatment of pain than any other form of analgesia, including analgesic drugs. Thus, for some patients acupuncture may be used as an alternative to analgesic drugs. In others, depending upon the cause of the pain, acupuncture may prove to be superior to available drugs; in yet other patients the converse will be true. In those patients for whom acupuncture is an effective form of analgesia it has the great advantage that it is devoid of the unwanted effects that can be produced by drugs.

Types and methods of acupuncture

Ordinary acupuncture is carried out by means of sterilized stainless steel needles, usually of 0.3 mm diameter (30 standard wire gauge, SWG) with a range of 0.1–0.4 mm diameter (42–27 SWG) and 10–60 mm (0.5–2.5 inches approximately) in length. Some classical acupuncturists also use silver and/or gold needles and may claim that these possess special qualities. In *superficial acupuncture* each needle is inserted to a depth of a few millimetres (Figure 14.1). The needle may then be left untouched until removed several minutes later or twirled for part or all of the time that it is inserted into the skin. In *deep acupuncture* the needle is inserted to a greater depth, sometimes with the aim of stimulating a specific deep structure, for example, the periosteum of a particular bony prominence, so-called 'periosteal pecking' by Dr Felix Mann. Naturally, the accidental piercing of a vital structure or organ must always be carefully avoided and therefore the practice of acupuncture demands a knowledge of the anatomy of the human body.

Other forms of Acupuncture: In addition to ordinary acupuncture there are other methods and systems of acupuncture that are used by

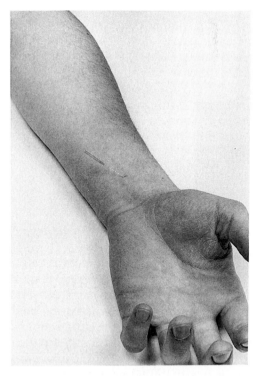

Figure 14.1 *Superficial acupuncture.*

different acupuncturists depending upon their training, the purpose for which the acupuncture is being used and also, to some extent, the part of the world in which they practise. Thus there is acupressure (finger pressure applied to acupuncture points); electroacupuncture (the passage of electrical currents through one or more pairs of needles inserted into acupoints) (Figure 14.2); moxibustion (applying a piece of ignited moxa plant *Artemesia vulgaris* to the acupuncture needle in order to intensify the stimulating effect); auricular acupuncture (a system of acupuncture applied to the external ear).

Uses and efficacy of acupuncture analgesia

Acupuncture is used to control many different types of pain and whilst it is often effective, unfortunately extravagant claims are sometimes made about its efficacy. In 1986 Richardson and Vincent carried out a critical review of the literature on studies that had been designed to measure the efficacy of acupuncture analgesia and at the same time they prepared another review of the methods used to evaluate the analgesia (Richardson and Vincent, 1986; Vincent and Richardson, 1986). On the basis of published work it appears that those painful

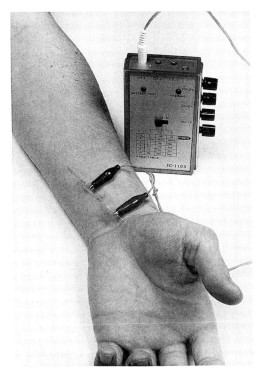

Figure 14.2 *Electroacupuncture.*

conditions for which acupuncture is most commonly used are as follows:

Main Uses:	Headache	C
	Back pain	C
Others:	Phantom limb	
	Sore throat	C
	Dental Postoperative pain	C
	Cancer	
	Peripheral neuritis	
	Rheumatoid arthritis (knee)	C
	Osteoarthritis (many sites)	C
	Cervical syndrome	C
	Bursitis and tendonitis	
	Mixed groups	C
	Facial pain	C
	Shoulder pain	C
	Post-herpetic neuralgia	C

C = Controlled studies carried out

Richardson and Vincent's survey of *un*controlled studies suggested that 50–70% of patients show a successful response which is much higher than would be expected on the basis of a placebo response which would be of the order of 30%. Their summary of trials on the efficacy of acupuncture for the treatment of back pain illustrates the variability of response even when the trials are controlled. Thus, the success rate with controlled trials for back pain varied between 26–79%, whereas those with uncontrolled trials reported a success rate of 47–82%. One of the factors responsible for the large scatter of results is due undoubtedly to the widely varying measures that were used to assess the analgesic effect of acupuncture. Nevertheless, one may fairly draw the conclusion that the majority of patients treated with acupuncture for back pain will derive clinically significant short-term benefit. Thus when all the results are taken into account it may be concluded that short-term relief is achieved in 50–80% of patients treated but the amount of long-term benefit achieved is not clear because 50–58% of long-term responders relapse. However, two important points must be remembered. First, it would be unreasonable to expect any form of treatment to result in everlasting analgesia unless the treatment has been able to eradicate the cause. Furthermore, patients who continue to respond to acupuncture can achieve prolonged pain control by undergoing repeated courses of acupuncture. Second, the situation is not essentially different from that where medication is used to control pain because analgesia is only maintained so long as medication is continued; once medication has stopped then pain is liable to recur.

Current theories on the mechanism of acupuncture with special reference to psychological effects

Acupuncture analgesia may be viewed as a situation in which a small pain is deliberately induced (the needling) in order to control a large pain (acute or chronic pain problem). It seems clear that it must switch on pain-relieving systems that are already built into the nervous system. The results of many different experiments suggest that acupuncture analgesia depends upon a number of mechanisms which operate at different levels of the nervous system. Thus, in ascending order, the peripheral nerves, spinal cord, mid-brain and probably higher centres of the brain are all involved. The first crucial step is the stimulation by needling of sensory nerve endings (A delta group) because acupuncture will not work if, for some reason, these nerves cannot function normally. In the spinal cord the arrival of needle-induced impulses activates local nerve circuits to release certain neurotransmitters and neuromodulators, including the endogenous opioids, which result in closing the so-called 'pain gate' (*see also* section on TENS; pages 171 and 176). In addition, signals are sent up the spinal cord to the mid-brain where additional nerve circuits are activated and which in turn activate certain *descending* nerve pathways. The latter which depend upon the release of certain other neurotransmitters, particularly serotonin (5-hydroxytryptamine), result in a widespread closing of pain gates at levels of the spinal cord above and below that at which the original needle-induced impulses entered. Thus these local (segmental) and distant (extra-segmental) effects of acupuncture would explain the traditional use of needles both close to and distant from an area of pain; for example, the use of acupoints on the scalp and foot for the treatment of migraine.

However, these mechanisms cannot account for one of the most useful and fascinating effects of acupuncture which is the prolonged analgesic action so often seen. Thus acupuncture analgesia can persist for several days or even weeks before further treatment is needed. On the basis of research carried out by Professor Han and his colleagues in Beijing, China, it seems possible that this prolonged analgesia is the result of acupuncture setting in motion a loop circuit between the mid-brain and limbic area of the brain. This loop of nerve activity, which involves the release of serotonin (5HT) and opioid peptides, blocks the passage of pain information to those centres of the brain where pain is perceived. It is postulated that this 'meso-limbic loop of analgesia' takes a long time to slow down, so accounting for the prolonged analgesic effect.

The relationship between acupuncture and psychology is two-fold. Thus there is the effect of acupuncture on the psychological responses of the patient to pain and conversely, the effect of the patient's psychological constitution on his or her response to acupuncture. It is well established that acupuncture raises the pain threshold but it seems likely that it also reduces the emotional response to pain in the same way as does morphine resulting in such comments from patients as 'Although I can still feel the pain, it does not upset me like it did'. Another important point which distinguishes acupuncture from TENS (*see* later) is that it provides an excellent opportunity for both tactile and oral communication between therapist and patient. Thus it combines both 'laying on of hands' and psychotherapy, each reinforcing the other. However, results of controlled clinical trials indicate that acupuncture does not work by psychotherapy alone. Furthermore, the effects of *electro*acupuncture may vary with the frequency of electrical stimulation used and this is probably due to the frequency-dependent release of those neurotransmitters responsible for the analgesic effect. Thus Han's work has shown that low frequencies elicit a relatively large release of an opioid peptide that acts on the same receptor as morphine, where it can be blocked by naloxone (a morphine antagonist). By contrast, high frequency stimulation causes the preferential release of different opioid peptides (as well as other unrelated neurotransmitters) that are probably less likely to alter the emotional response to pain. It is thus possible that low frequency acupuncture may be more effective in treating pain that is associated with a strong emotional component.

The psychological trait (personality) and state (mood) of a patient are also likely to influence the response to acupuncture via pathways that descend from the highest centres (cerebral cortex) to the mid-brain and spinal cord. Thus acupuncture may produce diametrically opposite effects on mood. After treatment, some patients experience euphoria whilst others feel relaxed and sleepy. Yet others may regularly feel nauseous and unwell for about 24 hours following which they recover and simultaneously experience excellent and long-lasting pain relief. These represent examples of so-called 'strong reactors' to acupuncture (a term coined by Dr Felix Mann) and illustrate well the importance of psychological factors in acupuncture.

The interaction between psychology and acupuncture may explain why severe depression is not usually helped by acupuncture. It could be argued that as severe depression may be associated with a deficiency in serotonergic mechanisms, this would explain the failure of depressive illness to respond to acupuncture. It should also be noted that schizophrenia does not usually respond to acupuncture.

Method of referral to an acupuncturist

Acupuncture is practised to varying degrees in all countries of Western Europe. In some countries, for example, France, Italy and Austria, acupuncturists must be medically qualified. In other countries, for example, Germany, Sweden and the United Kingdom, acupuncture can be practised by those who do not possess a medical qualification as well as by those who do. In the British Isles there is still much controversy as to whether it is desirable for acupuncture to be practised by non-medically qualified personnel but this issue will not be discussed here. Suffice it to say that acupuncture is an invasive technique and must therefore be practised using the highest possible standards of technique, including disposable sterile needles. Patients may be referred for acupuncture through a medical practitioner (if not already an acupuncturist) or may consult an acupuncturist directly. Names and addresses of local acupuncturists can be obtained by contacting the following addresses:

For Medically-qualified Acupuncturists:
British Medical Acupuncture Society
Administrative Officer
Newton House, Newton Lane, Lower Whitley, Warringon, Cheshire,
WA4 4JA. Tel. 092 573 727.

Non-medically-qualified Acupuncturists:
British Acupuncture Association,
34 Alderney Street, London, SW1V 4EU.
Tel. 071 834 3353/1012.

Transcutaneous electrical nerve stimulation (TENS)

Historical

The use of electricity for therapeutic purposes (electrotherapy) and particularly for the relief of painful conditions (electroanalgesia) goes back into antiquity. Thus, stone carvings dating from the Egyptian Fifth Dynasty made in approximately 2500 BC illustrate clearly the use of the electric fish (*Malapterurus electricus*) being employed to treat painful conditions! The electric torpedo fish was also known to Hippocrates in 400 BC who used it for the treatment of headache and arthritis. More recently, in the 18th century, physicians and surgeons employed electroanalgesia both to treat painful conditions and to produce surgical analgesia. In 1965 Melzack and Wall proposed a new theory concerning the mechanism whereby the nervous system controls the input and distribution of those nerve impulses which signal tissue damage and which, if directed to the higher centres of the brain, will be perceived as pain. They named this the Gate Control Theory of Pain, a fundamental corollary of which is that electrical stimulation of low threshold touch fibres should close the 'gate' and thereby block the onward transmission of impulses signalling tissue damage (nociception) and so obtund pain. Wall and Sweet (1967) soon showed that high frequency (50–100 Hz) percutaneous electrical nerve stimulation relieved chronic neurogenic pain. This fundamental discovery, coupled with the advent of solid-state electronic devices, resulted in the rapid development of portable battery-operated stimulators for pain relief. In 1973 Long reported that electrical stimulation could be applied via skin electrodes (Figure 14.3) thus establishing the technique of transcutaneous electrical nerve stimulation (TENS), the use of which has spread widely ever since for the treatment of different forms of acute and chronic pain.

Principles of use of TENS

Many different chronic pain conditions can be treated successfully with TENS which can also be used for treating some forms of acute pain, for example, postoperative pain. Numerous studies, including controlled clinical trials, have indicated that the *three* major factors,

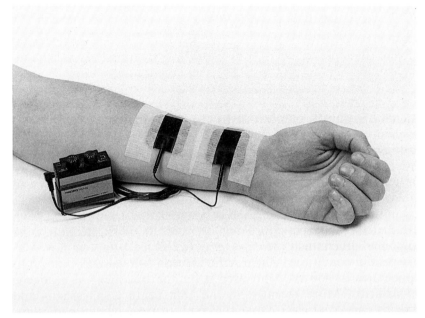

Figure 14.3 *Showing application of skin electrodes for TENS.*

which need to be considered when using TENS are the pain, the patient, and predictability of the response.

Pain

Pain can arise from one or more of five main sites: (i) superficial somatic, (ii) deep somatic, (iii) visceral, (iv) neurological, and (v) psychogenic. The question arises as to whether there is any correlation between the site of origin of a pain and its likely response to TENS? The results of clinical trials using TENS and also of extensive experience with it makes it possible to generalize and state that the likely effectiveness of TENS will be as follows:

1 Most effective—superficial somatic, deep somatic, neurological

2 Less effective—visceral, and

3 Least effective—psychogenic

These conclusions are obviously of great importance when considering the possible use of TENS for the treatment of a particular pain. For example, the pains following shingles (post-herpetic neuralgia), an amputation stump or an osteoarthritic joint are much more likely to respond to TENS than pain arising from chronic pancreatic disease (chronic pancreatitis) which in turn is more likely to respond than pain of psychological origin.

Patient

It has been clearly established that for a particular chronic pain problem (i) some patients respond to TENS better than others; (ii) some patients fail to respond to TENS, i.e. they are non-responders; (iii) some patients respond well initially and then fail to respond, i.e. develop tolerance to TENS. At the present time it is not known why patients with similar pain conditions respond differently to TENS but it is almost certain that the causes are multifactorial. When an initially good response rapidly dwindles within a few days the explanation is most likely to be due to a placebo response. A good response that continues for several months and then fades is likely to be due to some compensatory mechanism of the nervous system which at the present time can only be conjectured upon. However, it must be made clear that there are patients whose response to TENS is fortunately maintained indefinitely.

Treatment Plan

Experience in Newcastle and elsewhere has shown that the simplest way to find out whether or not TENS will produce effective pain relief in a particular patient is to loan a clinic stimulator for a trial period of one month. By this means it can be given an exhaustive test under everyday conditions of the patient's life during which time the patient is encouraged to experiment with different positions of the electrodes together with different types and duration of stimulation. During this trial period the patient is also encouraged to contact the clinic for any advice required and if the need arises to return to the clinic for further practical advice. The following are typical directions given to each patient:

'Begin with one hour three times a day'
'Adjust according to need'
'Use as much as you like'
'You may get a bonus of post-TENS analgesia' (i.e. the pain relief will continue for a varying period after the stimulator has been switched off).

Ideally, the patient should be reviewed at 3-monthly intervals during the first year of TENS therapy and thereafter reviewed according to need.

Complications and Contraindications

Two major advantages of TENS therapy are that the incidence of adverse effects is low and that there are very few contraindications to its use.

1 *Complications* Allergic reactions are uncommon but may occur and

are due to: (a) the electrode; (b) the jelly, or (c) the fixative, e.g. tape, gum, etc. This can usually be remedied by replacing the offending item with a suitable alternative. Occasionally an electrical skin burn occurs and is usually due to bad technique caused either by overenthusiastic use or by incorrectly applying the electrodes to an area of skin that has undergone partial or total sensory loss. The use of reputable equipment minimizes the chances of equipment failure although the leads are always the weakest link in the chain.

2 *Contraindications*: These are very few but are important and must be noted:

(a) *Danger of stimulating anterior part of neck*: Patients should be advised never to try to stimulate over the anterior part of the neck because of the risk of stimulating the carotid sinus thereby producing hypotension and/or stimulating the nerves to the laryngeal muscles and so causing laryngeal spasm.

(b) *Pregnant uterus*: Except when used for obstetric analgesia, TENS should not be used in the vicinity of a pregnant uterus because of the very remote possibility of inducing labour.

(c) *Interaction with cardiac pacemaker*: TENS equipment is liable to interact lethally with an on-demand cardiac pacemaker and so must never be used in conjunction with such equipment. Other non-demand cardiac pacemakers *may* be safely compatible with TENS equipment but before these two instruments are used together it is *essential* to seek advice from the respective manufacturers.

(d) *Non-compliant patient*: Occasionally patients will be encountered who have a congenital inability to handle any form of electrical equipment, including stimulators, or who have a rooted fear of using electricity for medical treatment. In some cases this is due to a low I.Q. or to senility. In all of these patients it is worthless to pursue the use of TENS.

(e) *Psychological pain*: For reasons discussed earlier, pain which is either largely or totally psychological in origin usually responds poorly if at all to TENS therapy. Occasionally, a patient whose pain is predominantly or totally psychological in origin does obtain a useful response from TENS by some mechanism which is not clear. In these instances it seems likely that the TENS is a 'channel' through which the patient is able to switch off some mechanism which generates the pain.

It should be noted that when a patient has been clearly established as suffering from psychological pain (predominant or total) it is not wise to suggest a trial of TENS as a method of treatment. This is because to do so suggests to the patient that there is a local physical cause for the pain which may well contradict all the previous advice given to the patient concerning the mechanism of his or her pain.

Furthermore, if TENS is given a trial and fails (not surprisingly) the patient will interpret this as being yet another unsatisfactory treatment for what he or she considers to be a physical condition and consequently will continue to search for other forms of physical treatment instead of accepting the psychological nature of the problem.

It should be noted that patients taking anxiolytic drugs or corticosteroids may show a reduced response to TENS. Conversely, patients on tricyclic antidepressants and tryptophan may show an enhanced response.

Forms of TENS commonly used

Two forms of TENS are commonly used. (i) Continuous TENS consists of an unbroken train of pulses at a preset frequency. (ii) Pulsed or 'burst' TENS consists of intermittent trains at about 2 Hz of pulses at a preset frequency. Evidence available suggests that these two forms of TENS activate different pain-relieving systems. Thus, the pulsed or 'burst' form of stimulation which is commonly used with a high intensity of stimulation is associated with the release of opioid peptides such as enkephalins and endorphins. By contrast, the continuous form of stimulation does not appear to involve the release of opioid peptides. Therefore, when advising a patient to use TENS for the treatment of a chronic pain condition, it is important to make sure that both forms of stimulation are given an adequate trial. Sjölund and Eriksson (1980) have shown that, on average, continuous TENS is effective in 25% of patients whereas pulsed ('burst') TENS is effective in 40–50% of patients. Therefore, both forms of stimulation should always be included in a trial of TENS before it is abandoned for some other form of therapy.

Stimulators available for TENS

The number of stimulators designed specifically for the application of TENS therapy has increased steadily during the past decade. In the Pain Relief Clinic at the Royal Victoria Infirmary, Newcastle upon Tyne, we have standardized on two instruments which have been found by our patients, nurses and medical staff to be effective, reliable, and economical. Each instrument is purchased by and remains the property of the National Health Service and is then loaned to any patient who requires a stimulator on the basis that it is to be returned to the clinic when no longer required. The stimulators used are the 'Tiger Burst' (R.D.G. Electro Medical) which has now been replaced by the second version of the 'Tiger Pulse' stimulator; the other is the 'Microtens 7757 S' stimulator (Neen Pain Management Systems). Since it is outside the scope of this chapter to discuss different stimulators in detail, the interested reader is referred to a useful and critical evaluation carried out by J.M. Stamp and his colleagues at Sheffield (Stamp, J.M. and Wood, D.A. comparative evaluation of transcutaneous electrical nerve stimulators (TENS) Part 1, 1981; Part 2, 1984. Sheffield, Sheffield University and Area Health Authority.)

Cost-effectiveness of TENS therapy

Compared with medication, TENS therapy possesses two major advantages. First, after the initial capital outlay, the running costs are low, especially because the stimulator will last for many years. Second, when a stimulator is no longer required by one patient the instrument can be issued to another (whereas a partly used bottle of analgesic tablets cannot be transferred to another patient but must, by law, be destroyed).

Predictability of Response

As discussed earlier, at the present time it is not possible to predict *with certainty* whether a particular pain condition in a particular patient will respond to TENS. Therefore, if the use of TENS is contemplated for the treatment of a particular patient, then the only way to find out whether or not TENS is likely to be effective is to give the patient a trial of this form of therapy. It should be noted that, in essence, this situation is no different from that when a patient is given a trial of an analgesic drug. However, where the situation does differ is that whilst the route of administration of a drug is simple (usually oral), the optimum route of administration of TENS therapy by way of skin electrodes must be found by trial and error and is therefore initially time consuming and requires patience.

Unfortunately, the latter is not always appreciated with the result that patients may be denied an effective—and sometimes the only— form of therapy.

Results of Treatment with TENS

Using present-day techniques and equipment, approximately two-thirds of patients respond to TENS therapy and one-third either fail to respond or become rapidly tolerant to it. Of the two-thirds of patients who continue to respond there is unfortunately a slow drop out over the next six months or so resulting in a residual core of about one third of the original number of patients who continue to respond to TENS indefinitely. Thus, the author has a substantial number of patients who have been using TENS effectively for over five years and some are now approaching ten years of use. It must be remembered that for many of the long-term responders, TENS therapy is the only means of controlling their pain. It is clearly of great importance to try to elucidate the mechanism of tolerance to TENS and also ways to prevent it, problems which are the subject of a research project in the author's laboratory.

Acknowledgements

The author wishes to thank Mrs Margaret Cheek for her conscientious bibliographical and secretarial assistance during the preparation of this chapter. He would also like to thank Mrs Valerie Wright for additional secretarial assistance.

Bibliography

Han, J. S., Yu, L. C. and Shi, Y. S. (1986) A mesolimbic loop of analgesia III. A neuronal pathway from nucleus accumbens to periaqueductal grey. *Asia Pacific Journal of Pharmacology*, **1**, 17–22

Long, D. M. (1973) Electrical stimulation for relief of pain from chronic nerve injury. *Journal of Neurosurgery*, **39**, 718–722

Mann, F. (1987) *Textbook of Acupuncture*. Heinemann, London

Melzack, R. and Wall, P. W. (1965) Pain mechanisms: a new theory. *Science*, **150**, 971–979

Requena, Y. (1982) *Acupuncture et Psychologie*. Maloine s.a., Paris

Richardson, P. H. and Vincent, C. A. (1986) Acupuncture for the treatment of pain: a review of evaluative research. *Pain*, **24**, 15–40

Sjölund, B. and Eriksson, M. (1980) *Relief of Pain by TENS*. English translation 1985. John Wiley, Chichester

Thompson, J. W. (1986) The role of transcutaneous electrical nerve stimulation (TENS) for the control of pain. In 1986 International Symposium on Pain Control (ed. D. Doyle), International Congress and Symposium Series. No. 123. Royal Society of Medicine Services Ltd, London

Vincent, C. A. and Richardson, P. H. (1986) The evaluation of therapeutic acupuncture: concepts and methods. *Pain*, **24**, 1–13

Wall, P. D. and Sweet, W. (1967) Temporary abolition of pain in man. *Science*, **155**, 108–109

15

Physiotherapy

L. M. Smith

Physiotherapists will be aware of the many manual techniques and therapeutic modalities which can be used in various circumstances to afford relief of pain (e.g. forms of heat therapy, electrotherapy, mobilization techniques, etc.) but such strategies are frequently inappropriate, or of secondary rather than primary importance in the management of the patient with long-standing chronic pain when there is psychological or psychiatric disturbance associated with pain. Long-term pain inevitably has effects upon the behaviour of the individual, and this in turn will influence the interactions of the individual with others. The physiotherapist cannot ignore the subsequent difficulties that arise from this change of behaviour.

Aims of treatment

The prime task of the physiotherapist is to improve mobility and function in all patients who are referred to him. Any improvement in these areas is of enormous importance to the patient with chronic pain who has lost so much of his previous abilities. There may well be considerable difficulties in achieving such aims when the patient has psychological or psychiatric problems associated with pain, but it is important that the physiotherapist remembers what is his main task and does not become side-tracked into talking at length about the patient's difficulties. This is necessary and important at the start of treatment but should not obscure the therapist's main task later which is to enable the patient to function more effectively in his environment.

Patients referred to physiotherapists from pain clinics are often not referred for pain relief as such, rather the physiotherapist is consulted as the expert who can determine, and perhaps alleviate the effects of chronic pain upon the musculoskeletal system and general mobility and lifestyle of the patient. The primary source of the pain in such patients may be, but is not inevitably, located in the musculoskeletal system itself, for long-standing pain from whatever source can have repercussions on mobility in its widest sense. Many patients misinterpret pain arising from infrequently used muscles and joints as evidence of further bodily injury and therefore refrain from carrying out any activity that causes any degree of pain. Muscle fibres shorten if not used and when stretched inevitably lead to an increase in afferent impulses which are often perceived as pain. As the pain felt by the patient is localized over the same area of the body that may have sustained the original injury, he is more likely to believe that the pain is due to the same cause as the original injury. Patients who misinterpret their symptoms in this way are more likely to have psychological and behavioural problems because of the considerable reduction in function that has occurred.

Evaluation of the problem

Referrals to the physiotherapist are normally made by other members of the pain clinic team. At the outset, the physiotherapist should be clear exactly why the patient has been referred and be clear about treatment goals. As much relevant background information as is available should be supplied by the team member making the referral. It is clearly preferable to attend the clinic with other members of the team and then these issues can be discussed face to face. This is not always possible, and if the physiotherapist normally works away from the pain clinic, it is more important that comprehensive written information about the patient is supplied. The ideal situation is referral, followed by a case conference about the patient with all professionals concerned.

Sufficient time must be allowed at the first appointment for a detailed evaluation of the patient's problems. It is useful to use a body chart to map the pain graphically, annotating the chart with a full description of the nature, intensity, frequency and behaviour of the pain and any other subjective symptoms (see Figure 15.1). The history of the disorder should be clearly understood, and the subjective assessment should elucidate a clear picture of how symptoms affect life-style. It is vital to assess the premorbid level of functioning and how the patient felt about himself and his body. Patients who have taken great pride in their body and physical activities are often disproportionately distressed when injury or disease alters function.

It is valuable to talk the patient through a typical day in his life and to question the patient on his relationships with significant others. The attitude and sensitivity of the therapist are all important during this initial session. Preconceptions on the part of the therapist must be avoided, questions must be 'open-ended', and the ability to listen to what is being said and to pick up on what is being inferred, are vital to the relationship which is established at the initial session. Objective measurements can then be made appropriate to the disorder. From the assessment as a whole, a clear picture should emerge of the patient's pain problem and consequences for the patient of living day-to-day with that pain.

The physiotherapist must then determine the problem from the physiotherapy perspective, and decide upon the attitude, approach and strategies which should be used to attempt to solve these problems. It is suggested that it requires a therapist with considerable clinical experience to deal sensitively and sensibly with those in chronic pain where there are psychological or psychiatric aspects to be considered. The inexperienced tend to focus on one particular issue which is usually of a physical nature. Unless the complex interaction of physical, psychological and behavioural factors is appreciated, the patient will not be sufficiently motivated to comply with the physiotherapist's instructions. Mason (1985) has emphasized that effective physiotherapy is not just the effective application of techniques but involves the recognition of the patient as a person. In what she calls her holistic approach, the individual is seen as more than the mere sum of his constituent parts. All the elements that contribute to his 'wholeness', whether they be physical, mental, spiritual, cultural, environmental or psychic must be considered. Mason further states that therapy must be capable of being directed towards any of these aspects of the individual, whether this is done overtly, or indirectly through the medium of attitudes, approaches, or strategies. The therapist should be prepared to adopt this holistic approach when dealing with patients with chronic pain when there are associated psychological or psychiatric elements, whether these elements predate the pain or whether they are a consequence of it.

Treatment strategies

Treatment approaches for the patient with chronic pain include the following procedures:

1 Information and explanation of origin of pain and maintaining factors

2 Change in treatment emphasis with transfer of responsibility to patient

3 Application of physiotherapeutic techniques, with particular consideration of behavioural principles.

Information and explanation of origin of pain and maintaining factors

Patients with chronic pain usually have some explanation about the origin of their pain. It is important to find out exactly what they believe the pain is due to and to correct any misapprehensions that they may have. It is often found that information provided by the doctor is not fully understood and may even serve to hamper treatment. Often the patient is more inclined to talk to the physiotherapist and he can act as an advocate in the bewildering liaison that the patient may have with senior professionals. The patient may ask 'what did the doctor mean when he said ... ?', and the physiotherapist is in an excellent position to educate and correct misunderstood information.

Change in treatment emphasis with transfer of responsibility to patient

Up until the time that the physiotherapist first sees the patient, the treatments given to the patient may not require his active involvement; he is a passive recipient of treatments supplied by others. One of the most fundamental messages that the physiotherapist can give the patient is that change in function can be brought about by the patient himself. This is usually the first time that the patient has been told this and, if he has sufficient faith in the physiotherapist's knowledge about his condition at this stage, he is more likely to accept that this is possible.

Application of physiotherapeutic techniques with particular consideration of behavioural principles

The selection of the particular physiotherapeutic techniques for treatment will depend on what is most important to the patient and what can be readily achievable. The emphasis should be on attempting to improve function in an area that the patient particularly wishes to improve. All approaches should be considered including modalities available for relief of pain if the therapist feels that these are appropriate. The patient should be instructed about which exercises and manoeuvres they should carry out and they should also be told what they must *not* do.

The physiotherapist first identifies targets that the patient should aim for. These should be readily achievable and be clearly described and understood by the patient. The achievement of these targets is facilitated by identifying the steps that are required to reach them. The emphasis should be on small steps in improving function and mobility. Treatment consists of both exercises that are carried out in the physiotherapy department and home programmes. These tasks should be made as simple as possible and should be carried out regularly and as frequently as feasible during the day.

It is important to coordinate the information obtained from the physiotherapy programme with the other pain clinic professionals, particularly if there are any medical factors which may be hampering improvement.

Involvement of spouse or significant other person

Initially, it is recommended that the patient is seen on his own and contracts are made between therapist and patient. If the spouse or partner is involved at this stage there may be confusion about each person's role. However, if there is no improvement to begin with and if there appears to be a lack of motivation, there may be an advantage in involving the partner early on in treatment. As the physiotherapist sees the patient less frequently towards the end of treatment, the spouse or significant other person with whom the patient has close contact, can often be an invaluable aide in prompting the patient to continue his exercise programme and other relevant homework tasks.

Cessation of treatment

Patients should be informed at the start of treatment how long any treatment is likely to last. This can only be a rough guide, but it is not possible for patients to attend departments on a regular basis for longer than a few months. In practice, there is not usually a great deal of difficulty in deciding when contact with a physiotherapist should cease. The patients themselves, if they have recognized the value of the treatment and have learnt what they are able to achieve themselves, usually make a decision at some stage that it is unnecessary to come up to the department at regular intervals. It is sometimes helpful if the patients are seen at annual or six-monthly intervals for follow-up but usually only one or two visits of this type are necessary.

At the time that the patient is last seen, it is often again helpful to underline the benefits of increased mobility.

Case history

The following case history is offered to illustrate the approach taken to one particular individual with a chronic pain problem with associated emotional difficulties.

Case Study – Mr A., aged 37

Mr A. is a married man with three children who used to work as a bus driver. Eighteen months before being referred to the clinic a workmate played a practical joke on him and pulled his chair away from him as he was about to sit down. The patient landed very heavily on the bottom of his spine, causing him much pain. At his local hospital he was seen by his own doctor and by a physiotherapist who manipulated his coccyx, giving only temporary relief of symptoms, as did hydrocortisone injections. He was diagnosed as having coccidynia at first attendance and was given a trial of transcutaneous coccidynia nerve stimulation (TENS) which appeared to ease his pain significantly initially, but when reviewed five months later he reported his pain to be more extensive.

He was referred to an orthopaedic surgeon, and to a neurologist, but neither was able to offer help in reducing his symptoms. It was noted that whilst there was a histrionic component to his pain behaviour, he was felt to have a substantial organic component to this as he had local signs of nerve damage and his pain was closely related to posture. He was referred to the psychiatrist but although there was some pain relief from antidepressants his mobility remained restricted.

The Newcastle Pain Relief Clinic organizes a series of Pain Education Classes to which the physiotherapist contributes. Mr A. was interested in the talk given by the physiotherapist and he was referred by the psychiatrist to her for individual attention.

A full evaluation was made of the patient's pain problem in terms of his symptoms, pain behaviour, clinical signs, posture and current lifestyle. Since his accident he had not worked. He was reluctant to sit and walked with the trunk flexed, with a stiff-legged gait. Prior to his accident he used to jog, and undertake body building, but following his injury his level of physical activity was reduced and he argued frequently with his wife and children. He felt considerable bitterness towards the man who caused his injury.

On a visual analogue scale (VAS) of 0–10 he evaluated his pain at level 9 most of the time. It was put to him that given his low level of activity and such a high pain level an increase in activity could only make his pain a little worse, whilst it may well serve to make his life more rewarding. It was also suggested to him that his poor posture and awkward gait might now in themselves be contributing to his pain and that correction of these might eventually reduce this. He was able to accept both these hypotheses as reasonable. He was therefore taught simple leg and trunk exercises, concentrating on good quality movement performed smoothly and rhythmically, which he could do on a regular basis at home. He was urged to increase his exercises only gradually as dictated by pain. He was instructed in postural correction in sitting and standing and encouraged to walk with a normal gait. In the department, interferential therapy was sometimes used at the end of an exercise session to ease the increased pain caused by exercise, and he continued to use TENS at home, which afforded him some reduction in the severity of his pain. A good rapport between patient and therapist was encouraged by the therapist adopting a sympathetic attitude and involving the patient in discussion about his moods, feelings, and relationship problems.

He made excellent progress in physical terms, steadily building up his exercise level and improving his posture and gait, and reported that he felt more cheerful and less 'disabled' as a result. However, it was clear that his inability to work, and the removal of not only his Public Service Vehicle driving licence, but also his licence to drive a car, which had occurred following his accident, were both contributing significantly to his depression. The psychiatrist, in conjunction with the Disablement Resettlement Officer, managed to obtain part-time work for him in a factory and this was a tremendous boost to his morale and served to dramatically improve his relationships with his wife and family. He reported that as a result of the job there were days when his pain was increased, but the beneficial effects of the job upon him were such that he was willing to tolerate this.

The physiotherapist wrote on the patient's behalf to the Drivers Vehicle Licensing Centre to request the return of his licence to drive a car, and this was reinstated subsequently to the patient's delight.

After 8 sessions with the physiotherapist over a 4-month period Mr A. was discharged with the proviso that he could contact her for help and advice at any time in the future. When asked to re-evaluate his pain level on discharge he reported that he still might have periods when his pain level was 9 on the VAS, but that these were less frequent than previously, lasted a shorter time, and were more tolerable as he felt so much more cheerful and fulfilled.

This case study is useful to illustrate the features of the physiotherapeutic strategy which contributed to the team effort to achieve a successful outcome for this individual. Perhaps the first point to highlight is that the patient himself, after listening to the physiotherapist's contribution to the Pain Education Class, expressed interest in seeing the physiotherapist. Many patients with chronic pain of musculoskeletal origin will have had courses of physiotherapy at an early stage in their disorder and are reluctant to accept that further physiotherapy might now prove beneficial if it was not effective before. It is important to tell the patient that whereas physiotherapy in the early stages of a painful condition would probably have been directed at treating the pain itself, the therapy at the chronic pain stage will have a different emphasis. No progress can be made with an individual who feels that he is being sent to see a professional without a clear hope of some perceived benefit from the encounter.

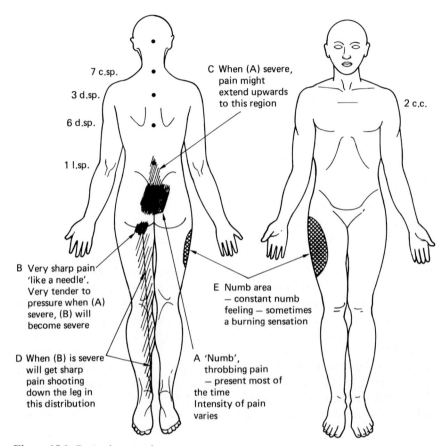

Figure 15.1 *Patient's pain chart.*

A detailed examination of the patient was conducted from the physiotherapy perspective; the patient's pain symptoms were charted (Figure 15.1) and it was made clear to the patient that the physiotherapist had a full understanding of the nature and severity of the symptoms. Patients are invariably reassured when the involved professional takes time to appreciate exactly what they are suffering.

Having understood and determined the patient's problems in discussion with the patient, problem-solving strategies were then also negotiated. It is suggested that there will be a greater patient compliance with treatment when the patient is involved in all decision-making processes. If the professional is willing to move away from the conventional professional/patient relationship characterized by control and management by the former towards a contract characterized by negotiation and equality, patterns of communication can be expected to alter greatly to the benefit of both therapist and patient. Mr A. responded well to such a strategy and worked hard on his exercise routine at home, often pushing himself beyond the level at which he was exercising comfortably to a point where exercise did indeed increase his pain. Most physiotherapists will have encountered the belief in certain individuals that they must make the pain worse in order to ultimately feel better. Because of the trust established between physiotherapist and patient, the deleterious effects of this behaviour could be discussed easily and Mr A. became more judicious in his homework exercises. At each therapy session the patient was encouraged to freely discuss his feelings. Achievements, however small, were praised, 'failures' made light of with the explanation that progress can rarely be expected to be a smooth continuum and he was not encouraged to discuss his pain levels as such but rather to congratulate himself upon any improvements in mobility, posture and gait.

It is suggested that an holistic approach by an experienced physiotherapist is a useful model for those dealing with chronic pain where there are psychological or psychiatric aspects to consider. A patient with severe psychological handicaps or psychiatric illness may rate his pain as high as possible (mark 10 on the visual analogue scale) and can, by definition, imagine no worse pain than he already has. If this pain results in severe restrictions upon his level of mobility, then it is possible to negotiate with the patient a therapeutic goal of improved mobility with the understanding that this will almost inevitably lead to a better quality of life with no increase in pain. It need not be made explicit at that stage that the psychological consequence of an improvement in quality of life often itself affects the extent of pain ratings. Increased function and mobility, coupled with the interest that can be developed when there is improvement in these areas, can have a pronounced effect on the patient's well-being.

Bibliography

Mason, A. (1985) 'Something to do with touch', *Physiotherapy*, **71**, 167–169
Saunders, H. D. (1985) *Evaluation, Treatment and Prevention of Musculo-skeletal Disorders*. Viking, Minneapolis

16

Organization of services in the pain clinic

J. E. Charlton

Introduction

This book has concentrated upon psychological and psychiatric aspects of chronic pain. However, any approach to the treatment of chronic pain which focuses on one or two aspects is unlikely to result in complete success. Indeed, given the complexity of chronic pain, it is probably unreasonable to expect an absolute cure in any case, except on the most rare occasions.

The treatment of patients with chronic pain has three distinct parts. Firstly, there is the effort to establish a diagnosis, and, where appropriate, treat the underlying cause. Secondly, there should be an attempt to assess the contribution of other factors, such as psychosocial problems, that may be increasing or perpetuating the pain. Finally, if the pain persists even after a full evaluation of the pain and management of any underlying disease or exacerbating factors, it is necessary to undertake symptom control. In other words, to treat the pain even though no previous therapy has been successful.

Many methods of pain relief are available and these range from conventional pain-relieving drugs and procedures which interrupt the passage of pain signals along nerves, to electrical nerve stimulators and strategies aimed at reducing the impact of pain upon the patient's life. Above all, the assessment must be comprehensive, painstaking and thorough with a special regard to intended therapy, which must avoid the potential for making the patient worse.

Patients with chronic pain have multiple problems. It is unreasonable to expect a single physician, no matter how gifted, to be able to understand, diagnose and achieve optimal treatment of all disease processes that may present as chronic pain. Thus the concept of the multidisciplinary pain clinic has been developed, where a group of specialists, all with an interest in the diagnosis and treatment of chronic pain, but with different specialist backgrounds, work as a team.

Pain clinics

These can take many different forms, and can vary from a multidisciplinary assessment centre to a single individual working in a hospital or office. In every case the aim is the same: to relieve or reduce pain using the safest and most effective methods possible. The pain clinic is frequently viewed as a last resort. The typical image of a pain clinic patient in the minds of both patients and doctors is either of an individual with terminal cancer who is racked with excruciating, unrelieved pain, or alternatively, a hopeless neurotic with persistent complaints involving every system in the body in whom no cause has ever been found. Pain clinics frequently are seen by members of the medical profession as convenient dumping grounds for patients whose complaints they cannot understand, or cannot be bothered to understand.

In general, pain clinics treat patients as outpatients or day cases. Inpatient management may also be offered as part of the pain clinic service.

The overall efficacy of a pain clinic is dependent upon it being multidisciplinary in its approach. This offers the opportunity to evaluate and treat all aspects of the pain complaint in an integrated fashion. Importantly, most patients are far more willing to accept psychiatric, psychological and social evaluation when this forms part of a multidisciplinary package that addresses their other complaints as well.

History of pain clinics

In the USA the first multidisciplinary pain clinic was pioneered by Dr John J. Bonica at the University of Washington, Seattle. This concept has been developed over thirty years and now serves as the model for all other pain clinics throughout the world. Dr Bonica has written extensively on this topic and has laid down several conditions that he feels are necessary for a successful pain clinic. Chief among these is the belief that each member of the group must have a special interest in pain and its relief. In addition they must be willing to devote time to gain the necessary knowledge, experience and skills in their own discipline. They must also acquire a broad knowledge of the basic and clinical aspects of disciplines other than their own. In other words they must be a good 'team player' with the ability to accept and use advice from other disciplines regarding the management of pain conditions.

In the UK and many other countries throughout the world, the treatment of pain has developed in a different fashion. Individuals, rather than multidisciplinary groups, began seeing small numbers of patients, and treated them with simple means such as drugs or nerve blocks. These individuals came from many disciplines, and frequently were anaesthetists; but this monospecialist approach inevitably restricted the assessment and treatment available to that which was within the training and expertise of the person running the clinic. This is not to say that this was wholly a bad thing, as these individuals rapidly acquired assessment and treatment skills outside their own disciplines and inevitably sought help from other consultants with difficult problems, this evolving a multidisciplinary approach, but without the formal structure of the American clinics.

What do pain clinics do

The purpose of a pain clinic is to diagnose and treat pain complaints. In addition, most pain clinics carry out teaching of doctors, nurses, students and other specialists in health care. They also carry out research into pain problems and evaluate new drugs, techniques and equipment. Pain clinics will treat patients as inpatients and outpatients according to need and facilities, and many will send specialists to see patients in their own home if this is necessary. Pain clinics have also developed close links with hospices and cooperate with palliative care physicians in achieving optimal pain relief for the terminally ill.

Diagnosis

A major purpose of any pain relief clinic is to establish a diagnosis in patients referred to it. Many patients are referred with vague or conflicting diagnoses, or even without diagnosis at all. Reasons for this apparent paradox can be found in conventional ways of treating disease and illness. A single specialist will make a diagnosis and institute treatment within the limits of his or her own knowledge and training. If that individual has no expertise in identifying a particular pain complaint, misdiagnosis and consequent mistreatment becomes a possibility. This may be a particular problem where the original specialist seeing the patient uses an invasive form of therapy as the first line of treatment, for example, surgery. The temptation for the unwary is to try an operation and see if it helps—all specialists, including surgeons, may be ignorant about other forms of treatment. 'When you've got a hammer, everything looks like a nail'. An inappropriate operation may lead to further pain complaints and compound the problems faced by the patient.

Thus, specialists of one discipline must always be most careful in their diagnosis, and not give opinions outside their area until the necessary expertise has been acquired. Despite this, a full discussion with the patient as to the diagnosis, or lack of it, may be of great benefit. Frequently patients have been misinformed or have misunderstood efforts to explain their symptoms and problems. It is always worthwhile discussing what are their concepts of the problem, as much of the hostility engendered by unsuccessful attempts to diagnose and treat pain can be reduced by good communication and mutual understanding of the issues.

Treatment

Many different therapies are possible, and some are outlined in earlier chapters of this book. However, much treatment may be instituted outside the confines of the pain clinic, and patients may be referred to other specialists. This brings us back to the concept of the multidisciplinary clinic where the skills of the individual can summate to form a whole, and this in turn makes the best sort of treatment for the patient more likely. The methods by which these services are organized will be discussed shortly. As mentioned previously, care must be taken to avoid any therapy that has the potential for making the patient worse.

Teaching and research

The fact that pain clinics exist is evidence that the majority of doctors know insufficient about painful conditions and their management. Teaching is not just a matter for health care professionals, but should also involve patients, as outlined in Chapter 13. Learning more about the reasons for pain has been shown to be of benefit in helping patients come to terms with a painful condition and adapting their lifestyle to accommodate it.

Larger pain clinics and clinics attached to medical schools will have training and teaching as part of their normal activity, but this applies to lesser degrees in all pain clinics. Similarly, research is an essential part of any endeavour in pain relief, and patients may have even done their own 'research' by sampling the effect upon their pain of 'alternative' therapies such as osteopathy, chiropractice or homeopathy.

Organization of pain clinics

Multidisciplinary pain clinics

These clinics require a director of clinical services who will be responsible for the overall administration and coordination of the activities of the clinic. This individual will be assisted by other clinicians who will act as the patient's managing physician or as a consultant. Consultants are other members of the pain clinic team with specialist interests and skills.

Each patient seen in the pain clinic has a manager who is responsible for their care during the period of their assessment and treatment. The concept of a patient manager is an important one and can be illustrated as follows. When the pain occurs for the first time, it is common for the primary care physician to assume, quite reasonably, that the pain is due to a treatable condition and prescribe treatment such as simple analgesics. Both patient and doctor often then assume that the passage of time will lead to resolution of the problem. If this fails to occur, a variety of tests may be ordered to try and ascertain a physical cause for the pain. If this search proves unsuccessful, the next step is to refer the patient for a specialist opinion. If the first opinion does not yield a diagnosis, a second is sought, and so on. This leads to fragmentation of care, poor communication and reinforces in the patient's mind the fact that something must be seriously wrong. Distress, uncertainty and emotional change may be a secondary result.

The next event may be a sudden and dramatic referral to a psychiatrist with the assumption 'that it's all in the mind'. However, the psychiatrist can frequently assure the patient that they are suffering from no mental illness, merely the effects of unrelieved pain, and the cycle begins again. Had a single individual taken on the role adopted by the patient manager in the pain clinic, the patient may have benefited more from seeing multiple specialists, and arrived at both diagnosis and understanding in a shorter time.

Without an individual taking responsibility for coordinating referrals, specialist opinions, and diagnostic tests, the patient can become lost in a merry-go-round of different specialists. This may lead to confusion of opinion, multiple medication and even unnecessary surgery. The patients may become angry and frustrated at the apparent lack of progress and anxious and depressed about its significance. This is not to say that patients do not benefit from this fragmented approach; many do, but there is plenty of evidence that suggests many would benefit more from a coordinated assessment of physical, psychological and social factors. In addition, most patients are more satisfied when dealing with an individual and will be able to accept suggestions for treatment more readily.

The doctors who work in pain clinics range widely in specialty, and may include anaesthetists, psychiatrists, neurologists, pharmacologists, orthopaedic surgeons and neurosurgeons as well as many other disciplines. In addition, important contributions are made by paramedical personnel such as clinical psychologists, physiotherapists and social workers. The emphasis which each clinic places on the care it offers will be a reflection of the number and specialty of personnel in the clinic. It is accepted convention that large multidisciplinary clinics (known as pain centres), will contain specialists from six or more different disciplines. This size of clinic is extremely rare outside North America.

There is no uniformity about the sort of specialist found in the clinics. Most pain clinics in the USA include anaesthetists, but have a high input from clinical psychology when compared to other countries. Outside North America pain clinics tend to be smaller and physician-oriented, often being led by anaesthetists. The emphasis upon clinical psychology probably stems from factors which are unique to North America where significant problems with drug usage may occur, and where pain clinics are funded by private health care schemes rather than state insurance, and the need to generate income has to be considered as a legitimate goal of the clinic. In his writings Bonica has stressed the necessity to avoid overemphasis of psychological factors and adopt a broadly-based approach. The multidisciplinary approach has one other advantage in dealing with a society and group of patients that are becoming increasingly litiginous. A law suit is much less likely to be successful when the treatment has been agreed by a group of specialists from several different disciplines.

Monospecialist clinics

These represent the simplest forms of pain clinic where a single doctor sees a small number of patients. The facilities available may be meagre and the range of conditions that can be treated by this sort of clinic will be limited. Treatment will be largely confined to one, or two areas, for example, drug therapy and, in the case of the anaesthetist-run pain clinic that is common in the UK and elsewhere, diagnostic and therapeutic nerve blocks.

Other pain clinics

In between the individual and the large multidisciplinary pain clinics are a wide range of other facilities. Some are small multidisciplinary clinics with smaller numbers of specialists than are usually found in the larger centres. These clinics will be able to carry out virtually every test or treatment, but may not perform certain complex procedures, such as neurosurgery. These clinics can be both 'open', and offer access to referral by any physician, or 'closed', and restrict referrals to physicians working in that hospital or health district. Certain pain clinics are syndrome-oriented and will see only patients with a specific condition or complaint. Examples would be clinics seeing back pain, headache or orofacial pain. Yet others are treatment-oriented and use a single therapy such as acupuncture or hypnosis to treat a wide variety of complaints. The disadvantages of this sort of approach are obvious.

Referral of patients

Referral to a pain clinic is usually by the patient's primary care physician or by another hospital specialist. This may be for treatment of a condition that is already diagnosed and for which an appropriate treatment is available in the pain clinic. Alternatively, it may be for assessment of other factors influencing the complaint of pain, or it may be for the purposes of establishing a diagnosis.

Regrettably, there are no predictors to determine which patients will benefit from referral to a multidisciplinary pain clinic. More unfortunately, such treatment is expensive, time-consuming and labour intensive, and many patients are not helped. Part of the problem is that we do not understand the complex mixture of physical and emotional problems that are found in chronic pain. Referral is probably appropriate where there appear to be both behavioural and physical reasons for pain, or where there are complex emotional and social problems or excessive drug intake.

In all instances the first job of the pain clinic physician is to review all known facts about the patient's problem. Ideally this should be contained in the referral letter, but frequently information is not available that will decide whether or not this is an appropriate referral to the pain clinic. This information can be obtained from careful review of notes, diagnostic tests and X-rays from previous admissions. With the initial appointment many clinics also send forms, questionnaires and activity diaries for the patient to complete prior to the first clinic visit.

On the basis of the referral information and review, a decision will be taken whether the patient should be seen initially as an out-patient, or whether admission is indicated. To a certain extent this decision will be taken in the light of how far the patient has to travel to the clinic as well as the patient's complaint and presentation. Extensive in-patient assessment and treatment programmes are almost unique to North America and are beyond the scope of this chapter. In-patient investigation and treatment may be undertaken elsewhere, but is usually on a limited basis, and solely for cases of unusual complexity or requiring specialist procedures. An exception would be in the case of simple pain management programmes which will be discussed later.

Assessment in the large multidisciplinary pain centre involves the taking of a history and a clinical examination by a pain clinic physician, not necessarily the patient manager, and frequently a member of the trainee medical staff. Psychological questionnaires and a full interview with a clinical psychologist, plus appropriate biochemical tests and X-rays complete the initial part of the assessment, which is then presented to the managing physician. This individual would then arrange consultation with other members of the multidisciplinary team. In practical terms the larger clinics work in much the same manner as smaller clinics and consultation is only arranged with specialists relevant to the patient's likely diagnosis. However, some clinics involve all the clinic staff in the assessment procedure, and this consultation process and subsequent case conference can be both time-consuming and expensive of consultant's valuable time.

In most smaller pain clinics the patient will be seen and examined by a physician who will assume responsibility for choosing and coordinating consultations within the pain clinic and with other specialists where appropriate. In the USA virtually every patient has an assessment by a clinical psychologist; in smaller clinics elsewhere an assessment of this sort is obtained only where indicated. The clinical psychology service runs parallel to the medical assessment, not in series. The omission of the case conference in the majority of cases permits better and more efficient use of consultant's time and the resources of the clinic. In addition, the physician's role as the patient's manager means they will act as liaison between the patient, the referring physician and the other members of the pain clinic. When all consultation has been completed, the physical findings and results of diagnostic tests are reviewed and a diagnosis and treatment plan are formulated. If this is straightforward, treatment can be undertaken in the pain clinic, or the patient can be referred back to the original physician with recommendations for future management. The small number of patients in whom the diagnosis or therapy are uncertain can be discussed at a conference of members of the pain clinic and a consensus achieved about the most probable diagnosis and treatment.

Staffing at pain clinics

Most pain clinics in the UK started with an individual, usually an anaesthetist, seeing patients on an occasional basis. There were no fixed facilities, and they made the best use possible of time and space not allocated to others. Modern pain relief requires, at minimum, two or three fixed outpatient sessions each week, with further sessions devoted to diagnostic and therapeutic procedures such as neural blockade, and to administration. Problems occur with this sort of clinic in the provision of pain relief services on occasions outside the time when clinics are being operated. In addition, there are further difficulties in covering absence due to sickness and holidays, providing cover for inpatients and running a consultation service. Pain problems do not go away merely because an individual is absent, they are there to greet his or her return and this places stresses upon individuals running such clinics.

Full-time pain clinics require two or more members providing a service every day of the week. This solves the problems of absence, permits an effective consultation service and allows cover to be provided for inpatients. This is of great importance where pain relief services are being provided for patients with cancer and terminal illness. Terminal care units are a special case, and can provide one of the most rewarding and appreciated services of a pain clinic. They are usually separate units with their own staff, and pain is not the only, or the major problem in these units, but it is appreciated by all if pain clinic personnel take an active role to provide advice and treatment. Close cooperation with members of the terminal care team over timing and choice of technique is mandatory.

In any painful condition the choice of pain-relieving measures available in smaller clinics will be dependent upon the discipline and training of the constituent members. Where more than one technique is suitable for the management of a particular condition this can be decided by discussion. It should be remembered that colleagues from other disciplines may require other specialist facilities within the pain clinic.

Central to the smooth running of any pain clinic are the secretarial and nursing staff. Secretarial help is of paramount importance, and if more than three outpatient sessions are being held each week, a full-time secretary is essential. This individual will act as liaison between patients and medical staff, book appointments and arrange facilities for special procedures such as nerve blocks under image intensification. In addition, there are the problems of locating records and X-rays and handling the heavy load of phone calls and correspondence that the average pain clinic engenders. A good secretary contributes greatly to the smooth running of the clinic and can provide valuable information about patients and their response to the pain clinic and the therapy they are receiving.

Trained and sympathetic nursing staff are another vital ingredient in the successful pain clinic. Not only do they perform nursing duties, but they may also administer questionnaires, instruct patients in simple exercise programmes and in the use of transcutaneous electrical nerve stimulators and other small appliances such as heating pads and vibrators. Tolerance, understanding and acceptance of the emotional difficulties of the patients are vital attributes. In addition, they also serve as a useful conduit between physician and patient; many valuable insights into pain problems have been gained from discussion with nursing colleagues.

It is important to hold regular meetings of clinic staff. Meetings of medical staff ideally should occur bimonthly and facilitate the smooth running of the clinic, promote the team approach and are good for the morale of all concerned.

Physical facilities

The pain clinic itself can be sited anywhere in the hospital, but several factors must be borne in mind. It must be readily accessible to a group of patients who may arrive in wheelchairs or on stretchers, and many of whom are elderly. Thus it should be accessible to ambulances and be relatively easy to find. Access to all areas and the toilets must be appropriately modified for the handicapped and wheelchair bound.

Ideally the clinic should be based on the treatment options that are being offered. As a minimum it should contain separate areas for consultation, examination and treatment. In all clinics where invasive procedures are carried out the treatment areas should be fully equipped for resuscitation with basic drugs and equipment including oxygen supply, intravenous therapy, tipping trolleys and monitors. Adequate provision must be made for recovery from any procedure which may be undertaken. The number of rooms needed will depend upon the number of patients seen at each clinic and the range and number of procedures carried out. Provision must be made for a waiting area for the patients, which can also be used for conferences. There must also be accommodation for the secretary, the nursing station and adequate storage for records and equipment. Psychiatric or psychological assessments require quiet accommodation which can also be used for relaxation training, hypnosis and as a place for the patient to fill in questionnaires.

Each pain clinic should have access to X-ray and to in-patient beds. The latter are necessary for assessment and treatment of more complex cases, those requiring invasive procedures such as neurolytic blockade, or the placement of long-term intravenous access or epidural catheters for pain relief in cancer. Beds are also needed for patients requiring behavioural modification programmes although these are rarely provided outside North America. These are considered next.

In-patient pain management programmes

Over the years pain patients can develop pain behaviours (Chapter 3) which can lead to a dogged and persistent sets of strategies for seeking additional help from the health and social services. These patients are both costly and time-consuming to manage and can monopolize health care resources to such an extent that the provision of care to others begins to suffer. Chronic pain also has a damaging effect upon family and friends who, in turn, may influence the patient's attitudes and make pain behaviours worse. In-patient behavioural modification programmes have been shown in several centres in North America to have a beneficial effect upon patients' activity levels, medication consumption and work record (*see* Chapter 9).

The task of these programmes is primarily one of education. The first step is to encourage the patients to adopt responsibility for their own care and well-being. The patient and all members of his or her family are involved in such programmes which aim to improve the activity and level of social functioning of the individual. This can normally only be done effectively on an inpatient basis as the patient needs to be removed from their home environment where they can control events around them. On admission, patients undergo baseline assessment for physical and occupational activities. Their requirement for analgesic and sedative drugs is also analysed. Over a subsequent four to six week period several treatment goals are set for both patient and family.

These include a programme of increasing function and activity which is achieved by daily physiotherapy and occupational therapy, with continual setting of targets. Synchronously, there is medication control and reduction using tapering doses of analgesic and sedative drugs, with suppression of pain behaviour and gait re-education where indicated. Once goals have been set, the patients are taught skills that aid them in controlling their own pain. These may include transcutaneous electrical nerve stimulation, relaxation techniques and self-hypnosis.

As well as learning to control their own pain, many patients have to 'unlearn' inappropriate pain behaviours. This is best provided in an inpatient milieu, but several successful programmes have been undertaken on a day-stay basis. For maximum benefit the patient needs to be in an atmosphere that restricts access to drugs, and provides encouragement for active behaviour such as exercise or positive involvement with others.

On completion of a pain management programme there is always the danger that any benefits achieved in such programmes may be lost when the patient returns home, so the patient's family must be involved throughout the programme. This is essential when the behaviour of the family may be contributing to the problems.

Conclusion

Pain clinics have evolved to fill a perceived gap in the provision of health care, and the multidisciplinary approach is the most appropriate as no individual or discipline can have sufficient knowledge and expertise to have all the answers. The team approach avoids over-emphasis of any particular type of treatment or approach which is inappropriate.

It should be noted that pain clinics do not diagnose correctly in every case, and do not have 100% success rates. However, improvement is greater than in clinics where physicians work alone. Pain clinics serve to broaden our knowledge about the presentation and treatment of a wide range of painful conditions, and act as a bridge between different disciplines for the improvement of patient care.

Bibliography

Bonica, J. J. (1976) Organization and function of pain clinics. In: *Advances in Neurology* (ed. J. J. Bonica), Vol. 4, Raven Press, New York, pp. 433–43

Bonica, J. J., Bendetti, C. and Murphy, T. M. (1983) Functions of pain clinics and pain centres. In *Relief of Intractable Pain* (ed. M. Swerdlow), Elsevier, Amsterdam, pp. 65–84

Lipton, S. (1986) Current views on the management of a pain relief centre. In: *The Therapy of Pain* (ed. M. Swerdlow), MTP Press, Lancaster, 57–78

Mushin, W. W., Swerdlow, M., Lipton, S. et al. (1977) The pain centre. *Practitioner*, **218**, 439–43

Swerdlow, M. (1978) The value of clinics for the relief of chronic pain. *Journal of Medical Ethics*, **4**, 117–126

Appendix

Pain diary used in the Newcastle pain relief clinic

NAME: _____

DIARY FROM: _____ TO: _____
           (DATE)

We would like you to complete this diary during the next week.
Fill out a page each day, preferably a little bit at a time, several times
during a day. Indicate the major activity you were doing within each
2-hour time block.

PLEASE EXAMINE THE EXAMPLE ILLUSTRATED OVERLEAF

In the activity section please indicate what you have been doing
during the time indicated. In the thoughts and feelings section write
down how you have felt during the period and what thoughts have
been going through your mind.

In the central column marked PAIN, please indicate the degree of
your pain during the period specified according to the scheme shown
below:

	slight	moderate	severe	
NO PAIN WHATSOEVER	0 1 2 3	4 5 6	7 8 9	10 WORST PAIN IMAGINABLE

DATE: 20th March 1989   INITIALS: Mrs SL

Time	Activity	Pain	Thoughts and feelings
12–2 am	Sleep		
2–4 am	Sleep		
4–6 am	Woke up at 4.15 am with pain and got up to let cat out	6	Felt half-awake and unreal – the pain-killers must have worn off.
6–8 am	Woke up half an hour before alarm	7	Worrying about Len's (son's) problem with his boss – it makes my pain worse
8–10 am	Made breakfast, woke family (burnt toast)	8	When the pain is like this I can't do anything right
10–12 am	Took bus to town, shopped in market. Bought flowers	6	Shopping took my mind off my worries
12–2 pm	Had lunch in town with Vera (friend) window-shopped	8	Enjoyed Vera's company at first but then had argument about her children's behaviour. Made me miserable. Pain awful
2–4 pm	Took metro home. Sat and did nothing	8	Brooded over my problems. I wish I'd never had the operation
4–6 pm	Collected Sara from school. Made her tea. Prepared Joe's (husband's) meal	7	Felt empty even though I did everything right
6–8 pm	Had meal with Joe and Len. Talked about moving	7	I wish he would listen for once to my point of view. He doesn't understand what I am going through
8–10 pm	Watched TV for $\frac{1}{4}$ hour after reading story to Sara	6	Wish my life was like these stories
10–12 pm	Crocheted shawl for niece's christening. Bed at 11.00 pm	4	Made good progress. Joe in a good mood and this helped me.

Index